Penguin Books

HEALTHY GUT GUIDE

Jill Thomas is a naturopath, herbalist and iridologist and runs Albert Park Naturopathic Centre, a busy practice in inner Melbourne. She lectured at the Melbourne College of Natural Medicine (MCNM) for five years and spent a year as the resident naturopath at a Melbourne radio station. She has won numerous awards for clinical excellence in nutrition and herbal medicine, and graduated as dux of her year at the MCNM. Jill is the author of *Revive: How to Overcome Fatigue Naturally*.

HEALTHY GUT GUIDE

NATURAL SOLUTIONS FOR YOUR
DIGESTIVE DISORDERS

JILL THOMAS N.D.

Penguin Books

This book is not meant to replace or supersede professional medical advice. Neither the author nor the publisher can be held responsible for claims resulting from information contained in this book.

PENGUIN BOOKS

Published by the Penguin Group
Penguin Group (Australia)
250 Camberwell Road, Camberwell, Victoria 3124, Australia
(a division of Pearson Australia Group Pty Ltd)
Penguin Group (USA) Inc.
375 Hudson Street, New York, New York 10014, USA
Penguin Group (Canada)
90 Eglinton Avenue East, Suite 700, Toronto, ON M4P 2Y3, Canada
(a division of Pearson Penguin Canada Inc.)
Penguin Books Ltd
80 Strand, London WC2R 0RL, England
Penguin Ireland
25 St Stephen's Green, Dublin 2, Ireland
(a division of Penguin Books Ltd)
Penguin Books India Pvt Ltd
11, Community Centre, Panchsheel Park, New Delhi-110 017, India
Penguin Group (NZ)
67 Apollo Drive, Rosedale, North Shore 0632, New Zealand
(a division of Pearson New Zealand Ltd)
Penguin Books (South Africa) (Pty) Ltd
24 Sturdee Avenue, Rosebank, Johannesburg 2196, South Africa

Penguin Books Ltd, Registered Offices: 80 Strand, London WC2R 0RL, England

First published by Penguin Group (Australia), a division of Pearson Australia Group Pty Ltd, 2007

10 9 8 7 6 5 4 3 2 1

Designed by Elizabeth Dias © Penguin Group (Australia)
Cover illustration by Bridgeman Art Library/Getty Images
Author photograph by Jodie Hutchinson
Typeset in 11/16.25 pt Sabon by Post Pre-press Group, Brisbane, Queensland
Printed in Australia by McPherson's Printing Group, Maryborough, Victoria

National Library of Australia
Cataloguing-in-Publication data:

Thomas, Jill.
    Healthy Gut Guide.

    Bibliography.
    Includes index.
    ISBN-13: 978 0 14 300522 3.

    1. Gastrointestinal system – Diseases – Popular works. 2. Digestive organs – Diseases – Diet therapy.
    3. Digestive organs – Diseases – Homeopathic treatment. 4. Naturopathy. I. Title.

616.30654

www.penguin.com.au

For Ann and Tom, for always being there

ACKNOWLEDGEMENTS

A sincere thank you to Sam, Caitlin and Sophie at my favourite cafe for their thoughtful attention to detail and quality – the pretty plates are truly appreciated!

· · ·

Every attempt has been made to acknowledge source material. The author and publisher would be pleased to hear from any source whose work has not been acknowledged.

The case histories I refer to throughout the book are those of actual clients I have seen over the years; however, their names and personal circumstances have been changed to protect their privacy and for reasons of client confidentiality.

CONTENTS

1 Introduction   1

2 The digestive system: Where is it and
  what does it do?   7

3 The brain–gut connection: Could our gut
  be a second brain?   19

4 Irritable bowel syndrome   29

5 Banish the bloat   44

6 Gut flora: Getting the balance right   55

7 Constipation: What's the hold up?   69

8 Diarrhoea: An explosive exploration   89

9 Adverse food reactions: Allergies, sensitivities
  and intolerances   102

10 Coeliac disease and gluten sensitivity   116

11 Leaky gut syndrome   127

12 Halitosis: The last bad breath   132

13 The importance of digestive enzymes and
   hydrochloric acid   140

14 How to overcome a sluggish metabolism   154

15 Inflammatory bowel disease   177

16 Peptic matters: Duodenal and gastric ulcers   186

17 Healthy Gut Guide solutions   197

APPENDICES

1 The role of enzymes in digestion   213
2 Complete digestive stool analysis (CDSA)   214
3 Seed mix   215
4 Artificial sweeteners: Are they safe?   216
5 Crispy tempeh with avocado and tahini dip   218
6 Homemade yoghurt   219
7 Probiotic supplements and antibiotics   220
8 Fibre figures   221
9 Meadowsweet: A friend of the digestive system   223
10 Standard elimination diet   224
11 Gluten-free elimination diet   225
12 Food challenge diary   226
13 Wheat sources   228
14 A guide to gluten   229
15 Protein combinations for vegetarians   230
16 How to make that (herbal) medicine go down!   231

   References   232
   Index   239

1

INTRODUCTION

'Now, good digestion wait on appetite, and health on both!'
— *Macbeth,* SHAKESPEARE

A pain-free abdominal region is our right. We should, ideally, be unaware of our stomach and gut regions. Sadly, this is not always the case.

I wrote my first book *Revive: How to Overcome Fatigue Naturally* because of the alarming number of patients who, in the privacy of my naturopathic rooms, admitted that they felt exhausted most of the time. Vying with fatigue for equal position as one of the most common health concerns are bowel problems and abdominal discomfort. Hence the subject matter of this book.

A complaint I frequently hear mid-way through a naturopathic consultation is: 'By the end of the day I look like I am seven months' pregnant, I feel bloated and uncomfortable and it doesn't seem to matter what I eat.' Or, from male clients who are generally not so forthcoming when discussing bowels matters: 'I feel like my digestion is sluggish and I need a good clean out.' What is going on in the gastrointestinal tracts (GIT) of a large percentage of the population? Why are so many of us experiencing real discomfort somewhere along the nine metres of our GIT? Symptoms can include bloating, constipation, abdominal pain, diarrhoea, gastric reflux, escalating food allergies, gut-related headaches – and sometimes all these symptoms are felt in one day. A painful, uncomfortable gastric mix, indeed.

Fortunately, the answer to many of these symptoms is found at the end of a knife and fork. That is, what we choose to put into our mouths (or else not put into our mouths) is responsible for a great deal of abdominal pain. Whether it is a case of incompatible food combinations, undiagnosed food sensitivities, nutritional deficiencies, insufficient fibre, an imbalance of gut flora or a plethora of other causes, we are largely in control of both the causes and, very positively, the solutions to our digestive complaints.

Many of us have some sort of preoccupation with our stomach or bowels. The *Healthy Gut Guide* will help you understand how your GIT works and show you what you can do to heal your digestive disorders. Let's not waste time experiencing gut discomfort of any description. Remember your right – a pain-free gastrointestinal tract!

Hippocrates (460–377 BC), the father of medicine, very wisely remarked, 'All diseases begin in the gut'. He wasn't wrong. Optimal health is intricately linked to a healthy gastrointestinal system. We can't have one without the other. It may be surprising to learn that the GIT works directly with the nervous system and the immune system; therefore, diseases of the GIT not only affect the digestion and absorption of nutrients, but may also result in poor immune function, predisposing us to repeated colds and infections, as well as decreasing our threshold to stress, making us emotionally vulnerable and overly sensitive.

Given the fact that the GIT, compared with other organs, is a fairly simple construction, it seems to give us an inordinate amount of grief. Gastrointestinal disorders have been a source of human misery since ancient times. Indeed, Hippocrates himself left detailed descriptions of intestinal obstruction and liver disease. Later, the Greek physician Galen (131–201 AD) offered some interesting ideas about the digestive process and gastrointestinal diseases, notably ulcers of the oesophagus and stomach and hardening of the liver.

Other than the lung, the GIT is the only internal organ in contact with the external environment. Into this long, twisting, relatively hollow tube a startling array of chemicals are placed and manufactured. The foods we eat, the hydrochloric acid, pancreatic enzymes and bile we manufacture, as well as our beneficial gut flora, must all co-exist in a relatively friendly manner to ensure a healthy and pain-free environment. This is not always an easy matter, particularly when we add into this delicate mix the impact our emotional state has on our abdominal regions.

Stress, anxiety and depression are all well-established causes of digestive discomfort – think ulcers, constipation, diarrhoea or bloating – and it is important to understand how our mental state affects the performance of our GIT. It is fascinating to note that the brain and stomach develop from the same part of the human embryo and even share some of the same neurotransmitters and hormones. Hardly surprising, then, that our emotional state has a direct affect on our gut. Common sayings such as 'butterflies in the stomach', 'sick to the stomach' and 'gut wrenching' are backed up by sound scientific fact!

The best strategy to adopt for a pain-free GIT is prevention. Be kind to your intestines.

Ten crimes against your gut:

1) insufficient fibre
2) insufficient water
3) incompatible food combinations
4) gulping and rushing meals
5) eating when stressed or anxious
6) not allowing time in the morning for a satisfactory bowel movement
7) too many 'dead', de-vitalised foods (compare the dead energy of a can of luncheon meat to the living dynamism of a carrot!)

8) insufficient raw, enzyme-rich foods
9) excessive stimulants, such as tea, coffee, alcohol or spices
10) overeating.

If you can own up to even one of these misdemeanors, chances are you have experienced gut pain at some point in your life. However, if you have been very diligent and answer no to all of the above, yet still suffer from GIT discomfort, the following conditions may be contributing to a less than ideal gut zone:

- food allergies and sensitivities
- leaky gut syndrome
- stress and anxiety
- coeliac disease
- Crohn's disease or ulcerative colitis
- intestinal parasites
- peptic ulceration
- imbalance or insufficient intestinal flora
- insufficient pancreatic enzymes
- inadequate hydrochloric acid (HCl) production.

Together we will examine the diverse range of factors that can contribute to gut discomfort, pinpoint the possible causes and then discuss ways of addressing them with diet, herbal medicine, lifestyle changes and stress management. The solutions are in your hands. By the end of this book you will not only be the proud owners of a pain-free gut, you will have enhanced your general health and wellbeing in the process. A double bonus!

2

THE DIGESTIVE SYSTEM:
WHERE IS IT AND WHAT DOES IT DO?

The digestive system consists of two main parts. Firstly, the gastrointestinal tract (GIT), also known as the alimentary canal, which is one long (nine metre) tube extending from the mouth to the anus. The GIT includes the mouth, pharynx, oesophagus, stomach, and the small and large intestine. The second group of organs that are part of the digestive system, referred to as assessory structures, include teeth, tongue, salivary glands, liver, gallbladder and pancreas.

As readers of *Revive* will recall, food is our source of energy, it provides all the nutrients (carbohydrates, proteins, fats, vitamins and minerals) required to make a unit of energy. When food is consumed, however, it is not in any state suitable for use as an energy source. The main function of the digestive system is to break down food into molecules small enough to enter our cells and be converted into energy. The GIT transports the food we eat from the time we pop it into our mouths through the digestion and absorption stage, right through to the elimination of the unusable end products. Peristalsis – the wave-like contractions of the muscular wall of the GIT – breaks down the food by churning it up, while enzymes secreted by cells lining the GIT break it down chemically. Finally, peristalsis propels the food along the tract and into the rectum for elimination.

An exploratory journey along the GIT – with side trips to places of special significance

MOUTH

Digestion begins in the mouth. This crucial part of our anatomy is formed by the cheeks, hard and soft palates (front and back portion of the roof of the mouth, respectively) and the tongue. The tongue forms the floor of the mouth. This is where the digestive road starts, and, sadly, for many, where digestive problems begin.

Our mouths are a temporary holding chamber for the chewing and mixing of food with saliva. Chewing triggers the production of our stomach's digestive juices. Not chewing sufficiently and allowing too little time for adequate secretion of our digestive enzymes, particularly those involved in carbohydrate breakdown, is the source of much digestive angst. But more about that later. Bear in mind that the strongest muscles in our body are found on each side of our mouth – the masseters. These obliging muscles allow us to bite with a force of 75 kg cm^2. So, there is no excuse for not chewing our food into small, digestive-friendly pieces. The thousands of taste buds located along the tongue's surface help us distinguish between sweet, salty, sour and bitter flavours. Our senses of taste and of smell, in response to food odours, also help to trigger salivation and the secretion of gastric juice in the stomach.

SALIVARY GLANDS

Our three sets of salivary glands, lying just outside the mouth, pour their secretions into ducts that empty into the mouth. Together they secrete about one litre of saliva a day. Saliva is 99.5 per cent water and the balance is made up of enzymes, salts and minerals, which are continuously secreted into the mouth. However, when food enters the mouth the saliva secretion increases; it lubricates, dissolves and the enzymes start the chemical breakdown of food. Each salivary gland supplies different proportions of ingredients to saliva. The parotid glands secrete mainly amylase, an important enzyme that initiates the breakdown of starches. Salivary amylase continues to act on starches for 15–20 minutes after the food has been swallowed, *before* the stomach acids inactivate it. Another enzyme found in the saliva is lingual lipase. This enzyme, which is also active in the stomach, helps to break down and digest triglycerides.

YOUR GASTRO-INTESTINAL TRACT (GIT)

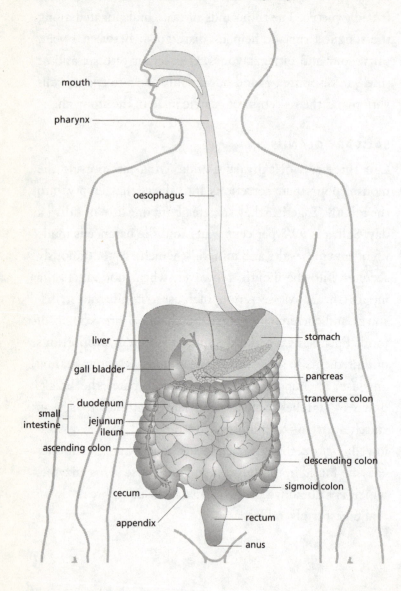

OESOPHAGUS

The oesophagus is a long muscular tube that connects the pharynx to the stomach. The connection between the pharynx and the oesophagus is controlled by a ring-like muscular valve called a sphincter; another sphincter is located where the oesophagus joins the stomach. The sphincter allows food into the stomach and prevents food refluxing back into the oesophagus. Through a series of wave-like contractions called peristalsis, the oesophagus delivers our now chewed-up food (bolus) into the stomach.

STOMACH

The stomach is a J-shaped, bag-like structure, and when empty it is roughly the shape of a large sausage – or in vegetarian parlance, a small cucumber. It begins at the bottom of the oesophagus and ends at the pyloric sphincter, which joins the stomach to the duodenum, the first part of our small intestine. It is interesting to note that the stomach actually sits to the *left* of the sternum, and not, as is often assumed, found mid-centre of the upper abdominal section.

The stomach is essentially a mixing bowl; it secretes digestive juices, mixes and stores food until broken down, and then propels partially digested food into the small intestine. Food, as it arrives, is stored in vertical layers in the upper section of the stomach (the fundus), until it is moved to the lower section where it is mixed and churned up. Fluid, however, passes relatively quickly through the stomach. The fruit salad you had for dessert, being mainly water, will pass quickly, while meat, being a dense protein containing very little water, will sit in the stomach for hours (which explains our feeling of fullness after a meal high in animal protein and fat). Hence this naturopath's constant nagging about *not* mixing animal proteins and fruit at the same meal. Unwise food combinations, such as this, will result in fermentation, which can cause bloating (see Chapter 5, Banish the bloat).

The stomach wall is lined with a thick coating of mucus – the mucosal barrier – which protects it from the digestive acids. The quality and quantity of this mucus together with the tight junctions formed by the cells of the stomach, make our stomach lining relatively impermeable to acid. However, aspirin, alcohol, regurgitated bile, nutritional deficiencies and food allergies can cause inflammation and ulceration and break down this important protective barrier.

GASTRIC SECRETION

Specialised cells in the stomach secrete large volumes of gastric juice composed of: mucus (which coats the mucosal lining, protecting it from damage), hydrochloric acid (HCl), potassium chloride, enzymes, hormones and intrinsic factor (necessary for the absorption of vitamin B12). HCl and pepsinogen are the most important gastric secretions.

HCl dissolves food fibres, acts as a bactericide and converts pepsinogen to pepsin (pepsin breaks down protein). Important to note that some ulcer medications suppress HCl production.

The presence of HCl in gastric juice was established by an English physiologic chemist William Prout, in 1824, by what must have been a rather uncomfortable procedure. Sponges were swallowed and retrieved, and the juice was then squeezed out and studied. Swallowing linen bags or perforated metal tubes filled with food allowed analysis of gastric digestion. Thankfully we have moved on from such scientific experiments, necessary but definitely not nice.

SMALL INTESTINE

This is *the* major site for the digestion of food and the absorption of nutrients. The duodenum, jejunum and ileum (which sit together in a rather compressed, coiled-up manner) make up the five metres of our small intestine. (The small intestine is a bit of a misnomer since the large intestine measures 1.5 m, in comparison.) Small finger-like projections, called villi, line the small intestine, greatly increasing its absorptive surface area. The villi absorb nutrients and secrete some of the enzymes necessary for digestion. Poor nutrition (especially a vitamin B12 deficiency), stress, drugs and irradiation suppress cell division, which shorten the villi and reduce their capacity to absorb nutrients.

The digested food (chyme) moving from the stomach into the small intestine, which has already been partially broken down by HCl and pepsin into food fibres, stimulates the liver and gallbladder to deliver bile and the pancreas to deliver enzymes. Carbohydrates are broken down into glucose and fructose, proteins into amino acids and fats are emulsified into fatty acids (see Appendix 1, The role of enzymes in digestion). These digested substances or nutrients, together with water, vitamins and electrolytes, are absorbed across the intestinal wall and then transported to the liver where they are further metabolised. The residency time of nutrients is crucial to the efficiency of absorption.

It is reassuring to know that the entire cell-wall lining of our small intestine is replaced every four to seven days. Hence, when undertaking a program of gut repair we can be assured that a damaged, leaky intestinal wall is quite capable of regenerating, given the right environment and healing substances (see Chapter 11, Leaky gut syndrome).

LARGE INTESTINE

The large intestine, which encircles the rather bunched-up small intestine, is made up of: the cecum, plus or minus our appendix (depending on its behaviour and any meetings with surgeons along the way), the colon – ascending, transverse, descending and sigmoid (the last section where the large intestine meets the rectum), and the rectum. The internal and external sphincters connect the rectum to the anal canal (the last port of call). This 1.5 m of tubing can give us enormous discomfort if all is not in tip-top condition – constipation, diarrhoea, diverticulitis, wind . . . need I go on?

The contents of the small intestine move into the cecum through the ileocecal valve, which prevents reflux into the small intestine, and are propelled along the rest of the colon by peristalsis. By this stage in its journey, the food, which we have chewed, digested, broken down and absorbed key nutrients from, is called the faecal mass. Increased volume and pressure in the sigmoid colon triggers peristalsis and forces the faeces into the normally empty rectum. This stretches the wall of the rectum and relaxes the rather uptight anal sphincter, creating the urge to have a bowel motion. We can override this urge by voluntarily contracting the external anal sphincter and pelvic floor muscles. This reduces tension, relaxes the rectal wall and the urge to defecate passes; however, repeatedly overriding this need to use our bowels can result in chronic constipation. Attending to the need to go to the toilet at the very moment it is experienced and not putting it off until later is a crucial habit to cultivate, if we are to achieve a constipation-free zone. (See Chapter 7, Constipation: What's the hold up?, for some useful bowel habits to follow.)

The large intestine is a treasure chest of bacteria (think bifidobacteria). Intestinal floras eliminate toxic bile by-products, convert unabsorbed carbohydrates into absorbable organic acids, are involved in the metabolism of oestrogen and androgens, lipids, as well as numerous nitrogenous substances and drugs. A minor imbalance in this precarious inner world of our intestinal flora population can result in major gut discomfort, not to mention serious nutritional deficiencies.

An important role of the large intestine is the absorption of water. It is also responsible for a great deal of fermentation – not the beer type but just as capable of producing the pot-belly look if out of balance. It provides the ideal environment for microbial fermentation of soluble fibre, undigested carbohydrates and starch. This in turn produces short-chain fatty acids (SCFAs), which are the main energy source for the epithelial cells of the colon. The short-chain fatty acids formed from this fermentation together with amines (the result of protein degradation) also help create the slightly acidic pH of faecal matter.

The large intestine is a hard-working member of our GIT and not, as Elie Metchnikoff, the nineteenth century Russian scientist, would have us believe, 'an asylum of harmful microbes . . . a source of intoxication from within'. Although, I have a sneaking suspicion there are still some members of the public who erroneously assume this to be the case, evidenced by their comments that they need 'a good clean out'. Metchnikoff's solution to this source of 'autointoxication' was surgical removal of the large bowel. A rather drastic approach to this indispensable part of our anatomy!

Assessory organs

LIVER

With regard to our digestive system, the liver produces bile for the absorption of fats, chemically breaks down amino acids (proteins), and is a storage receptacle for vitamins B12, A, D, E and K, and the minerals iron and copper. The liver is *the* great detoxifier, breaking down drugs, chemicals, pesticides and hormones found in the food chain. A ceaseless worker which, given the right conditions, rarely gives up.

GALLBLADDER

This is a small organ located just at the back of the liver and attached to it by a small duct. While the liver is the manufacturer of bile, the gallbladder is the storage shed. When food, especially fatty food, enters the small intestine, the gallbladder contracts and releases bile into the lumen of the small intestines. The bile salts emulsify and absorb fats, including cholesterol.

PANCREAS

The pancreas secretes pancreatic juice into the duodenum – the small tube connecting the stomach to the small intestine. This fluid neutralises stomach acid, and also contains digestive enzymes that break down carbohydrates, proteins and fats. The pancreas has another role, which is equally important and life sustaining: it produces insulin and other hormones that help maintain blood-sugar levels and ensure the effective uptake of glucose at the cellular level.

Given the above facts, being mindful of every single iota of food that we place in our mouths is of *paramount* importance. What we eat, when we eat it, what we eat with it and how we eat it are all crucial factors in determining the state of our guts and, indeed, our total wellbeing. Armed with our knowledge of the GIT, let's look more closely at some of the problems that can be encountered along the road in this part of our anatomical world.

3

THE BRAIN–GUT CONNECTION:
COULD OUR GUT BE A SECOND BRAIN?

'In the abdomen there exists a brain of wonderful power
maintaining eternal, restless vigilance over its viscera.
It presides over organic life . . . it is the centre of life itself.'
— The Abdominal and Pelvic Brain, DR BYRON ROBINSON

Our gut and brain develop from the same part of the
human embryo and share many of the same nerve endings,
hormones and neurotransmitters; thus ensuring a perma-
nent link between the brain and gut. Neurotransmitters
carry information from one nerve cell to another enabling
the brain and gut to send and receive messages. This relay-
ing of information affects everything – from blood flow
and abdominal muscle contraction to mental acuity.

The enteric nervous system (ENS) is the largest part
of our peripheral nervous system and controls digestive
processes. It has often been described as a brain in its
own right. It is truly amazing to discover that the ENS
can function independently of the central nervous system

(CNS). All of the key neurotransmitters found in the brain, including serotonin, enkephalin, histamine, substance P (which is released from the brain in response to stress, and stimulates a perception of pain), noradrenalin and acetylcholine can be found in the ENS. Anti-depressant drugs, such as selective serotonin reuptake inhibitors (SSRIs), cause gut-associated side effects because they increase serotonin levels in the brain *and* the gut. Serotonin in the gut initiates responses such as nausea, vomiting and the peristaltic reflex. Consequently, nausea and diarrhoea are often experienced when taking these medications.

Our emotions can also have a significant impact on the physiological functioning of our gut. Biochemical messages travel back and forth between the brain and gut in fractions of a second. The physiological effects of anxiety, for example, are palpable. We have all experienced the nausea and/or diarrhoea, sweating palms, rapid heartbeat, dry mouth and hyperventilation that are unpleasantly associated with feelings of extreme anxiety.

A whole new world of understanding gut disorders is at our fingertips once we get our heads around this vital connection. Let's thresh out this business of shared neurotransmitters between the gut and the brain a little further. Enkephalin, for example, which you may be familiar with in terms of its impact on our mental state through exercise, is also an important gut neurotransmitter. Its major action in the gastrointestinal tract (GIT) is to relax the smooth muscle and decrease secretions from the intestinal mucosa. However, as a significant CNS endorphin (there are three classifications of endorphins, enkephalin being one of them), it is responsible for our general sensations of wellbeing. It also inhibits pain transmission making it an indispensable analgesic, more potent and longer lasting than morphine. (Indeed, morphine and heroin bind to enkephalin receptors on nerve cells.) Stress, strenuous exercise, acupuncture and sex increase the levels of circulating endorphins. Therefore, as a protective mechanism, in appropriate circumstances, our brain directs our gut muscle to relax and reduce the production of key enzymes. However, if we have a gut disorder and our production of enkephalin is reduced, this will have a significant negative impact on our feeling of wellbeing, pain perception and mood. It works both ways.

Serotonin in the brain influences mood and cognition, and, as mentioned, also acts as a GIT neurotransmitter. Approximately 80 per cent of the body's serotonin is found in the gut, spreading itself throughout the entire GIT. Serotonin triggers vital gut reflexes; for instance, when an unwanted bacterium enters the gut, serotonin is released, which stimulates intestinal secretions, jump starts peristalsis (resulting in a bowel motion) and initiates nausea and vomiting. Not particularly comfortable responses, but brilliantly designed to get rid of unwelcome bacteria visitors. So next time you have a touch of food poisoning, give a little thought of thanks to your serotonin neuro-transmitter – it is working in our gut's best interests!

This brain-to-gut communication is undeniably crucial, and, naturally, a dysfunction in this neurotransmitter will affect GIT motility – not a pleasant thought. Now let's consider what the effect would be if serotonin levels are low. Several studies have linked low levels of serotonin with depressive and gastrointestinal symptoms. In regard to the GIT, insufficient serotonin may result in delayed gastric emptying, low levels of gastric acid and enzymes; symptoms could include constipation, bloating, dyspepsia, fullness and upper-abdominal pain.

So it is crucial to consider the state of our chemical messengers when addressing gut disorders. There is no point, for example, increasing levels of hydrochloric acid (HCl) to resolve symptoms of bloating and burping, if our levels of serotonin are low, for, as we have seen, this neurotransmitter regulates gastric secretion; i.e. HCl and enzyme production.

Stress and the gut

If we are what we think and what we eat, imagine the trouble we can create when eating incorrectly and thinking inappropriately. Why does eating in a state of anxiety undoubtedly result in gut pain?

Stress is an individual physiological and emotional response by our body to a demand that exceeds our own unique coping abilities. It is a non-specific response to any stimuli that requires us to change or adapt in some way. The way in which stress affects us depends upon our sensitivity to stress, the severity of the stress and the length of time we have been exposed to it. A stressor may be physical (heat, cold, a bleeding wound), chemical or biological (pollutants, food additives) or psychological (relationships, work pressures). Feelings that are experienced when stressed include anxiety, depression, irritability, exhaustion, oversensitivity and anger.

No matter what the cause, however, the impact of stress goes far beyond our feelings. As Hans Selye, discoverer of the general adaptation syndrome (GAS), noted: 'Every stress leaves an indelible scar, and the organism pays for its survival after a stressful situation by becoming a little older.' Research shows that even though feelings of anxiety may originate in the brain, the physiological effects cascade throughout the body. Stress and anxiety can lead to many physical changes: the thymus and lymph glands, responsible for our immune response, atrophy; the adrenal glands become enlarged and bloodshot; and the gastric mucosa become spotted with bleeding ulcers. Therefore, during stressful periods in our lives, not only do we become adrenally exhausted and have difficulty fighting infection, but we also experience escalating digestive disorders and gut discomfort. Stress can also do a fairly good job at wearing away our intestinal lining, resulting in leaky gut (a permeable gut wall) and all the associated systemic problems related to that; such as food sensitivities, fatigue, abdominal discomfort and bloating, joint and muscle pain and even headache and skin eruptions (see Chapter 11, Leaky gut syndrome). Anxiety and stress are also considered to be significant contributors to the conglomeration of symptoms that are given the umbrella term irritable bowel syndrome (IBS). (IBS is put under the microscope in Chapter 4.)

How does stress cause bowel discomfort?

- promotes gut inflammation
- increases gut permeability
- increases substance P activity
- alters secretion of gastric juice and enzymes
- increases mucus release
- decreases friendly bacteria (lactobacillus and bifidobacteria)
- increases opportunity for 'bad' bacteria to flourish.

A recent exciting discovery shows that changes in gut flora in IBS sufferers alters the content of neurotransmitters (NT) in the colon, resulting in an altered perception of gut pain. (Remember that substance P is a key neurotransmitter regulating pain perception.) In other words, an insufficient level of beneficial bacteria has a detrimental effect on our level of neurotransmitters in the gut, thus lowering our threshold of pain. This means that any distention or spasm in the gut will cause far more pain than normal. Even at the best of times the alimentary canal responds acutely to distention and spasm, which can be caused by physical blockage, irritants, wind or psychological factors. A decreased population of gut flora has also been linked to increased susceptibility to depression. Indeed, the link gets far more intriguing: 30 per cent of patients with major depressive disorder (MDD) suffer from IBS, and a prior exposure to antibiotic use (which wipes out the good bacteria as well as the bad) has been shown to be a risk factor in the onset of IBS with a major depressive element. Crohn's disease, an inflammatory bowel disease, has also been linked to depressive disorders.

However, no need for despair. Remember, we are in charge and nearly all damage is repairable. Not only do we have the means to undo any stress-created gut problems, but we also have at our fingertips the means to handle stress effectively to ensure no physiological damage occurs in the first place.

Treatment for a healthy gut–brain connection

Here are some guidelines to follow:
- Ensure correct nutrient levels to encourage adequate manufacture of the key neurotransmitters. Many neurotransmitters require co-factors such as: the amino acids

phenylalanine, tryptophan and tyrosine; vitamins B1, B2, B3, B5, B6, folate and vitamin C, plus the minerals calcium, magnesium, chromium and zinc. (As we have seen, low levels of the neurotransmitter serotonin result in constipation and bloating, so the priority in treatment would *not* be laxatives or peppermint capsules, but appropriate nutritional supplements to encourage serotonin production.) Do not self-prescribe these supplements, getting the right blend is crucial. Seek your naturopath's advice.

- Take a high-dose vitamin B complex, together with vitamin C and magnesium to support adrenal gland function. These nutrients are swiftly used up during periods of stress.

- Acute abdominal pain can be treated with a therapeutic dose of magnesium. It is best to take as a 200 mg supplement of magnesium orotate and magnesium aspartate three times a day. During acute attacks, take the cell salt magnesium phosphate (Mag Phos) every ten minutes until pain resides. Bromelain (a digestive enzyme found in pineapple) can reduce substance P and induce a significant reduction of the inflammatory pain cascade. Take 600–1000 mg a day.

- Bach Rescue Remedy is an ideal fast-acting

homeopathic remedy for acute anxiety; especially
recommended for the mouth-drying, heart-
pumping, nausea-making symptoms of extreme
nervousness and fear. Four drops on the tongue as
often as necessary.

- Treat underlying stress with a nervine herbal
  tonic. Herbs to consider (best prescribed by your
  naturopath) include: oats seed (*Avena sativa*);
  skullcap (*Scutellaria laterifolia*); vervain (*Verbena
  officinalis*); chamomile (*Matricaria recutita*) and
  lime flowers (*Tilia europa*), which is especially
  good for abdominal pain and nausea. For chronic
  stress the best herbs to use are Siberian ginseng
  (*Eleutheroccus senticosus*), withania (*Withania
  somnifera*) and gota kola (*Centella asiatica*).
  These herbs, known as adaptagenic herbs, protect
  and restore the nervous system, increasing our
  resistance to stress.
- Supplement with probiotics, notably lactobacilli
  and bifidobacteria, to replenish reduced beneficial
  gut flora. Take a capsule that contains at least 25
  billion cells twice a day before meals (see Chapter
  6, Gut flora: Getting the balance right).
- Deep abdominal breathing exercises help control
  rapid, shallow breathing. Yoga, meditation or
  Pilates are ideal ways to learn and perfect your
  breathing techniques.

- Exercise. Many studies support the mood-enhancing effect of exercise (think endorphins and enkephalins), and intense aerobic workouts are now used to treat depression and anxiety. Find an exercise you really enjoy and make it a non-negotiable part of your daily routine. (One of my clients reports that Bollywood dancing has a high belly-laugh factor as well as being an intense aerobic workout!)

4

IRRITABLE BOWEL SYNDROME

The term irritable bowel syndrome (IBS) makes me very grumpy. It tends to be used by those who should know better to describe a range of gut symptoms which the practitioner finds too tiresome or difficult to diagnose accurately. It is really just an umbrella term used to cover a diverse number of symptoms, including abdominal pain and altered bowel function, whose cause is not related to a specific health concern, such as appendicitis, gastric ulcer or gallstones.

Over the years I have seen many, many clients who have come to me after being 'diagnosed' with IBS, which later we found to be, in fact, multiple food allergies, leaky gut syndrome, spastic constipation, lactose intolerance, coeliac disease, stress-related bowel distension or inflammatory bowel disease (IBD).

In other words, they have a specific abdominal or gut-related problem that has rather shabbily been given a general diagnosis. Hence my irritation with the term irritable bowel syndrome! Of course these poor patients have an irritable bowel; they have serious gut problems that need *specific* treatment.

Here is a typical text book example of IBS: 'Irritable bowel syndrome is a common, debilitating, multifactorial, functional, gastrointestinal disorder where a definitive aetiology has not been established and no uniformly successful treatment exists. Diagnosis is now usually based on symptoms meeting the Rome II criteria.'!

The Rome II criteria, which sounds more like a papal directive than a clinical criteria for diagnosis, specifies that at least three months of abdominal pain, either continuous or recurrent, should be accompanied by at least two other symptoms. That is, pain is relieved by defecation and/or is associated with either a change in the frequency or consistency of the stool. And furthermore, if the patient is less than 45 years of age and meets three or more of the Rome II criteria, a confident diagnosis can be provided without the need for invasive testing.

So, in other words, if you had abdominal pain and a change in bowel habits, you are likely to end up with a diagnosis of IBS. This is not particularly helpful. Surely it is more important to treat the cause of these distressing symptoms rather than provide a diagnosis based on a tick-box method criteria?

Signs and symptoms of IBS

IBS is estimated to bother as much as 20 per cent of the population. This means a great number of people are wandering around with very uncomfortable abdominal regions. Indeed, IBS is believed to be responsible for 30–40 per cent of all gastroenterology appointments. Let's look at the signs and symptoms that will frequently result in an IBS diagnosis:

- abdominal pain, usually relieved by defecation
- diarrhoea or constipation, often alternating
- bloating
- flatulence
- loss of appetite
- nausea
- mucus in the stool
- gastric reflux.

These symptoms can often be accompanied by fatigue, poor sleep, backache and urinary problems, as well as depression and anxiety.

Diagnosis

The first step is to determine the cause. A thorough case history, dietary analysis, tongue, nail and iris examination are the diagnostic tools of the naturopathic trade, that, in most cases, provide me with the clues I am looking for.

Further investigations to be considered, if necessary:

- food-allergy blood test
- intestinal permeability urine test
- liver- and thyroid-function blood test
- lactose-intolerance test
- fructose-malabsorption breath test
- coeliac disease blood test
- stool analysis
- colonoscopy
- elimination and challenge test.

Treatment will depend on the outcome of the above investigations, and may include dietary and lifestyle changes, herbal medicine, vitamin and mineral supplementation, probiotics and exercise.

Causes of IBS

In my experience the major causes of IBS-like symptoms, in descending order of frequency, are as follows:

- inappropriate food choices and food combinations
- food allergies
- stress-related bowel distention
- insufficient fibre or the wrong type of fibre
- leaky gut syndrome
- lactose intolerance
- fructose malabsorption
- eating too quickly and/or when anxious
- altered intestinal microflora and/or small

intestinal bacterial overgrowth (SIBO)
- impaired tolerance of intestinal gas (In some people, the perception of pain associated with a distended intestine appears to be altered, so that 'normal' intestinal activity is felt differently.)
- bacterial infection of the intestine
- Crohn's disease
- parasitic infection, such as *Dientamoeba fragilis* or *Blastocystis hominis*.

Most of these conditions are discussed in depth in other chapters of the book, so, rather than repeating myself, let's look at some common triggers of an irritated bowel:
- fatty or spicy foods (especially where diarrhoea is a dominant symptom)
- excessive wheat bran
- coffee, tea and alcohol
- fizzy drinks
- sulphur-containing foods and additives
- artificial sweeteners and MSG
- smoking
- eating too quickly and not chewing thoroughly
- eating when stressed
- antibiotics, pain medications and anti-depressants
- food intolerances and sensitivities; especially to dairy, fructose and wheat.

Treatment for IBS

Most people who experience some of the symptoms gathered under the IBS umbrella, will have a tendency to either constipation or diarrhoea. And although these two symptoms may fluctuate, there is a discernable trend to experience one more than the other. So, in cases where *constipation is dominant* and the tone of the intestinal smooth muscle is too tense, probably in spasm, the following supplements and measures should be taken:

- magnesium
- aloe vera extract
- liver- and gallbladder-stimulating herbal medicine
- flaxseed meal
- bifidus probiotic
- exclude all tannin-containing drinks, such as red wine or tea (tannin causes contraction of the mucous membranes and reduces mucous secretion).

Where *diarrhoea is predominant* and the tone of the intestinal smooth muscle is too relaxed, the following supplements and measures should be taken:

- slippery elm bark powder
- astringent herbs; such as meadowsweet, agrimony or bayberry
- sip herbal teas between meals; such as peppermint, chamomile or lemon balm
- delete dairy foods

- delete caffeine and alcohol (stimulants speed transit time of food in the large intestine)
- *Lactobacillus acidophilus* or *Lactobacillus plantarum* probiotic.

Regardless of whether there is a tendency to either constipation or diarrhoea, a general treatment for IBS symptoms would involve the following supplements and measures:

- eliminate foods that contain sulphur, such as beans, broccoli, brussels sprouts, cabbage, cauliflower, garlic and onion
- eliminate carbonated drinks and chewing gum
- chew slowly and eat in a relaxed manner
- implement stress management techniques, if required
- eliminate high-fructose foods, especially apples, pears, onions, honey and wheat
- eliminate dairy
- eliminate coffee and alcohol
- ensure adequate intake of soluble fibre (introduce slowly, with small incremental increases in quantity)
- supplement with magnesium, a good-quality vitamin B complex, and short-term use of pancreatic enzymes and HCl
- herbal medicine (as prescribed), especially peppermint, chamomile, globe artichoke, fringe tree cramp bark, ginger and dandelion root

- probiotics, especially *Lactobacillus plantarum 299v*. Studies have shown that this strain reduces inflammation of the gut wall.

CONVENTIONAL DRUG THERAPY FOR IBS

Conventional treatment involves the prescription of antichol-inergics to treat gut spasm, diarrhoeals to stop diarrhoea, laxatives for constipation and anti-depressants for associ-ated anxiety and depression. An unappealing mish-mash of drug therapy that only treats the symptoms, which (once the treatment is stopped) will leave the poor patient in just the same gut-irritated state as when they began.

....

Let's look at two patients who came to see me with an IBS diagnosis; both suffering from pain and discomfort in the gut region but, as we shall see, from very different causes. And there have been many Susans and Rebeccas.

• • • •

Susan is an intelligent, vivacious woman in her late 30s who leads a very busy lifestyle: a demanding career, two young children, one with a learning disability, and is also actively involved in her local community, regularly holding open-house nights with live music and readings. She is on the go all the time, talking and moving at a lightning pace – her energy levels maintained by pure adrenal power (not good over the long term). Susan has frequent episodes of diarrhoea and nausea, alternating with the occasional bout of constipation, seemingly unconnected to her diet. Over the years she has tried a number of exclusion diets, with little improvement to her symptoms. She is often bloated, especially in the upper-abdominal region, and uncomfortable, complaining that 'by the end of the day I look nine months' pregnant'. Susan's gastroenterologist had sent her for a fructose-malabsorption test – a breath test that is performed at a few major hospitals – which had been positive. However, much to Susan's disappointment, a fructose-exclusion diet had had little impact on her symptoms (see page 113, 'Fructose malabsorption'). Her doctor felt there was little else to be done, and diagnosed IBS aggravated by fructose consumption. Hmmm. Before requesting further investigations, I asked Susan to keep a comprehensive diet diary for two weeks, noting symptoms against particular foods. I also prescribed a dairy-free acidophilus supplement as an interim measure to provide some temporary relief.

An analysis of Susan's diary indicated that dairy was strongly connected to her morning nausea, and that onions seemed to be a significant problem as well. Onions are very high in fructose. However, there were other worrisome symptoms seemingly unconnected to the usual dietary culprits of lactose and fructose. This made me especially suspicious of the presence of multiple food allergies and a leaky gut. I was concerned that Susan was not absorbing key nutrients, since, despite a reasonably well-balanced diet, she looked tired, had dark circles beneath her eyes and her nails had entrenched vertical ridges. (A sign of either poor absorption, lack of HCl, calcium or silica.) I ordered an intestinal permeability test (IP) and a food-allergy blood test. This was not a case for exclude and challenge. Susan had been suffering for far too long, and I doubted we would ever be able to ascertain all her allergies with a general food challenge.

As I suspected, Susan's IP test did not come back with an elephant stamp! Good and bad news, really. Naturally no one wants to discover they have a leaky gut, but then again better to know than not to know, and at least it was a definitive answer. In fact, Susan's IP test result was one of the worst cases I have ever seen of a porous intestine. Just as importantly, Susan's food-allergy blood test confirmed what we suspected – a dairy sensitivity – as well as enlightening us further with the startling news that she had allergic reactions to rye, peanut and the cola nut; that is, Coke. These food allergies had without doubt contributed to the high degree of permeability in her gut lining. Susan's past history of smoking (fortunately, she had given up 15 years ago) and her nightly glass or two of wine with dinner had also had a fair go at wearing away the intestinal lining.

We now had evidence that Susan had a mild degree of fructose intolerance, a number of food allergies and a very leaky gut. The answer was to exclude all the offending items and begin an intense course of gut repair. I could not prescribe one of our naturopathic powdered glutamine and licorice root supplements for gut repair as one product contained apple pectin, which contains fructose, and the other supplement was sweetened with fructose; so I prescribed pure glutamine in tablet form, to be taken twice a day with a ¼ cup of aloe vera juice before meals. This would rapidly repair the mucosal damage. I asked Susan to increase her water consumption by 500 per cent! She was in the very bad habit of drinking only two glasses of water each day. (The rule for calculating your daily individual water requirement is 35 ml water per kilo of body weight. That'll get many of you reassessing your water intake!) I felt that Susan's nervous system was severely stretched, and was concerned that this was exacerbating her diarrhoea and nausea; therefore, to strengthen her adrenal glands I prescribed a herbal supplement that contained the herbs Siberian ginseng and withania, as well as vitamins B5, B6 and vitamin C.

In our first consultation Susan had mentioned to me that she could remember episodes of diarrhoea occurring more than 20 years ago, after a trip to Africa. This immediately alerted me to the possibility of parasitic infection, so I asked Susan to have a stool analysis to rule this possibility definitely in or out (see Appendix 2, Complete digestive stool analysis).

Within six weeks of taking the glutamine, Susan noticed a definite improvement in her bowels. The bloating and odd 'worm-like' sensation in her upper-abdominal region also subsided. Fortunately her stool analysis was all clear, and

I should mention that a recent colonoscopy and gastroscopy were also both fine. I asked Susan to make a huge effort to increase the calcium in her diet because she was slightly built with a fine bone structure (in other words, a potential candidate for osteoporosis), and she had noticed that her hair had thinned over the past three months. She was to eat plenty of unhulled tahini, almonds, fish with bones and leafy greens on a daily basis. I gave Susan a calcium supplement to take at night (two before bed) to address the hair loss, but also to help her sleep as she had a long history of poor sleep patterns.

Although the stool analysis had proved negative – no unwelcome visitors lurking about – it did show evidence of undigested food in the stool. In Susan's case, this was more likely due to eating too quickly and when anxious than any intrinsic lack of pancreatic enzymes or hydrochloric acid (HCl); however, this provided a reason to persuade Susan to **slow** *down. I asked her to concentrate on eating, and chew each mouthful thoughtfully and thoroughly. I added to her treatment protocol a relaxing herbal mix of oats seed, lemon balm, vervain and lime flowers, which would have the twofold benefit of relaxing the central nervous system (CNS) as well as eliminating any spasm in the bowel. This was the turning point. After four weeks on this herbal mix, the diarrhoea ceased, nausea did not return, bloating completely subsided and the occasional glance in the toilet bowl assured Susan that she was digesting her meals thoroughly.*

I kept Susan on this herbal blend for a total of six months, and then prescribed a daily high-dose multi-vitamin to protect the adrenal glands and nervous system. We repeated the IP test after six months of gut repair, and, much to our relief, this time it returned with an elephant stamp! All healed.

....

Rebecca, a 27-year-old graphic designer, came to see me with a frustrating case of intermittent constipation, together with bloating and occasional lower-abdominal pain. Her doctor had diagnosed IBS and had prescribed some peppermint oil-based medication, designed to ease abdominal pain and relieve wind. This was not having a signicant impact on any of Rebecca's symptoms.

She had noticed in the past that whenever she was away on holiday she often missed a bowel movement; indeed, several days could pass without one. However, more recently, particularly since her partner had moved in, constipation had become a regular pattern, and to her dismay she was now only emptying her bowels, at best, every other day. Rebecca's constipation was strongly associated with stress. That is, it was a spastic constipation (spasm in the large bowel) rather than an atonic type (too little fibre, poor bowel tone). This is quite a common complaint amongst many of my female clients. (Interestingly men's bowels don't seem to be so affected by changes to routine or circumstance.) Lack of privacy and unpleasant lavatory facilities can cause stress-related abdominal pain and constipation. For example, how many of us can relax sufficiently in the tiny confines of an airplane toilet, which is used by at least a hundred others, to have a satisfying bowel motion – particularly towards the end of a 26-hour international flight, when conditions are, shall we say, a little stuffy?

I went through Rebecca's daily diet with a fine toothcomb and made a few fibre-enhancing changes. That is, instead of toast and Vegemite or a bowl of processed cereal for breakfast, I recommended a few tablespoons of seed mix with fruit and yoghurt or a high-fibre sugar-free muesli with a couple of tablespoons of linseed, sunflower and almond meal (LSA) (see Appendix 3, Seed mix). This was to be chewed very thoroughly and in a stress-free environment – **not** on the way to work in the car and **not** at the work desk! I also asked Rebecca to start her day with a glass of warm water and lemon juice in order to kick-start the liver. Otherwise, Rebecca's diet was quite well balanced – she ate a good range of fruit and vegetables plus legumes and beans, and drank sufficient water (1½–2 L a day). Rebecca's only other dietary misdemeanor was too many carbonated drinks; that is, flavoured mineral water or Diet Coke (see Appendix 4, Artificial sweeteners: Are they safe?). They had to go. Pouring carbonated drinks into a delicate stomach is not recommended. Gaseous bubbles do not guarantee a bloat-free abdominal environment.

I prescribed a magnesium supplement to relax the gut muscles, a vitamin B complex to soothe the nervous system, and herbal medicine to gently stimulate the liver and gallbladder.

I also asked Rebecca to allow herself sufficient time after breakfast to have a bowel movement. And she was to chat to her partner about giving her a little more personal space.

At the first follow-up consultation, two weeks later, Rebecca was feeling considerably better. Her bowel was more regular, now only skipping the occasional day; her bloating had reduced and her abdominal pain had virtually disappeared. Needless to say, she was feeling a lot less anxious – remember the connection between the gut and the brain. By the six-week mark, Rebecca was having a complete bowel motion daily and the bloating had completely resolved. I kept Rebecca on the herbal medicine for a three-month period, and encouraged her to eat plenty of bitter greens and maintain her lemon-in-warm-water-upon-awakening regime, which would gently stimulate any sluggish-liver relapses. Since Rebecca had a habit of holding stress in her gut, she maintained the magnesium supplementation for a further three months, and took up yoga with plenty of deep-diaphragmatic breathing.

....

Never accept the vague, 'let's put it in the too hard basket' diagnosis of IBS. As you can see there *is* a specific trigger or cause for your own unique set of gut symptoms. And with a little time, effort and perseverance these factors will be uncovered, ultimately rewarding you with a pain-free abdominal region.

5

BANISH THE BLOAT

One of the most frequently voiced abdominal concerns is bloating. Time and time again I hear the following complaint from my clients: 'When I wake up in the morning my stomach is reasonably flat, but by the end of the day it is horribly bloated and uncomfortable.' A distended, painful abdomen should not be the way in which we greet or, more commonly, end each day. Ideally, our gastrointestinal tract (GIT) should be getting on with its job without disturbing our peace and quiet.

Sadly, most people are at war with their stomach, and this state of affairs is due mainly to what we put in there. We should think of our stomach as a chemical laboratory, subject to the same scientific laws of action and reaction. If we fill it up, often at a single meal, with incompatible foods we are bound to end up with a gaseous, gurgling fermenting mass. Not very comfortable!

How is gas produced?

Gas is produced in the large intestine when fermentation occurs during the breakdown of certain carbohydrates and proteins. It is a normal by-product of the digestive process; however, too much gas causes bloating.

The daily production of gas in the GIT is between 500 and 1500 mL, with the volume at any given time being approximately 200 mL. Most of the gas responsible for flatulence (except oxygen) is produced by the 400-odd species of bacteria that live in our large intestines, including methane-generating, carbohydrate-fermenting bacterium. The average person passes between 500 and 2000 mL of wind each day. Oxygen is introduced by swallowing air during eating and drinking, or else through hyperventilation, which is often due to anxiety. Chewing gum, eating quickly or smoking will also increase our gaseous volume – unless it is expelled with a belch (preferably not in public).

Different foods can produce different amounts of gas. We are more than aware of the unfortunate effect of eating beans and legumes; however, a less well-known fact is that whole grains (raffinose), and fruit, onions and wheat, which are high in fructose (remember Susan), also produce a gassy by-product.

Sulphur-containing foods are also extremely gaseous. These include the brassica family of vegetables (also referred to as cruciferous) – broccoli, brussels sprouts, cabbage, cauliflower and turnip – as well as onions and garlic. Meat that contains sulphur in the form of food additives (e.g. sulphur dioxide and sodium metabisulphate) is also a dietary source.

The windy effect of beans and legumes can, to some degree, be lessened by cooking your beans with a small amount of seaweed (e.g. wakame, arame or kelp) or a few bay leaves. Be careful not to make the mistake I once made by thinking more is better, and adding a few generous strips of wakame to my pot of boiling kidney beans, only to find I had a steaming mass of seaweed pouring over the top of the saucepan within 10 minutes. Seaweed *expands* – cooks beware!

Causes of bloating

Bloating, like irritable bowel syndrome (IBS), has many causes; however, the most likely explanations are:

- small intestinal bacterial overgrowth (normally associated with diminished levels of microflora and insufficient enzyme production)
- imbalance of gut microflora
- food allergies
- lactose or fructose intolerance
- liver sluggishness
- eating in a hurry or when anxious.

Some of the common triggers of bloating include:

- foods that contain yeast, such as white bread, Vegemite and pizza
- raw, hard-to-digest vegetables, such as capsicum, carrot, onion and *unpeeled* cucumbers
- beans and legumes
- dairy foods
- carbonated drinks
- incompatible food combinations, such as melons or grapes with cereal and milk, and double proteins (e.g. ham and cheese)
- too many sulphur-containing foods, such as the brassica family of vegetables
- too much fibre or the wrong choice of fibre. (For example, psyllium, a fibre supplement, causes bloating and abdominal pain for many people. It must be taken with *plenty* of water and on an empty stomach.)

Don't panic about the length of this list of potential 'bloaters'. It is unlikely that all items will be a digestive problem for you; however, consider each one carefully and then cross it off the list if you can positively say it does not cause any digestive distress. If, after adjusting your diet and lifestyle to eliminate any likely bloating factors, you still experience abdominal pain and discomfort, then it's time to visit a naturopath to explore other potential factors.

Finally, I need to get something off my chest. No

charcoal tablets! Charcoal is for drawing with or burning, not for human consumption. Taking charcoal tablets to soak up excess gas will result in a seriously uncomfortable case of rebound constipation. If you have any charcoal tablets in your nutritional medicine cabinet, please throw them away immediately!

....

Clare's first words to me were, 'When I get up in the morning my stomach is completely flat, but by mid-afternoon most days I need to undo the top button of my skirt or pants as my stomach is hard and bloated. By the time I get home from work each night, I look and feel as if I am nine months' pregnant.' To illustrate the point, she lifted her top and showed me what was, indeed, a distended lower-abdominal region. Clare was tall and slim and her bloated stomach certainly did not accord with the rest of her frame.

Clare was 36 years old and has been suffering from the same complaint for at least 15 years. She had a colonoscopy 10 years ago, which was, fortunately, all clear. Clare also had a history of ovarian cysts, but her gynaecologist felt confident the abdominal pain was not related to this. A recent ultrasound supported that opinion. (I must say, I am constantly amazed at what some of my clients put up with. Never 'get used to' or 'live with' a health concern. There is always an answer.)

Clare had a reasonably healthy lifestyle, she exercised

regularly, did not drink tea or coffee and consumed alcohol only occasionally. However, she travelled extensively for work and, although her water consumption was adequate when on holidays or at home (1½ L a day), she confessed to drinking only a couple of glasses of water a day when travelling or on days that consisted of meeting after meeting. Clare had recently started drinking soft drinks as a mid-afternoon pick-me-up on work days, and had also experienced an uncharacteristic loss of appetite. Clare suffered from chronic constipation, having a bowel motion every couple of days at best, and at worst once a week. This definitely contributed to her discomfort.

When Clare described to me a typical day's diet, I easily identified a few potential 'bloating' factors. How many can you identify?

At breakfast, Clare had either toast and Vegemite; Weet-bix with psyllium, milk and fruit (usually watermelon or cantaloupe); or baked beans on toast; followed by a hot chocolate drink at mid morning. Lunch consisted of either a ham-and-cheese white bread roll or a Nori roll, and mineral water.

When dining at home, Clare cooked grilled steak or chicken plus a salad of lettuce, capsicum, onion, carrot and unpeeled cucumber or stir-fried vegetables, mainly broccoli, onion, cabbage, capsicum and bean sprouts. If out for dinner, fish, pasta or steak were the usual choices. Clare had takeaway about twice a week, usually pizza or Thai vegetarian curry.

After carefully going through Clare's diet, we agreed to make a few amendments: banish all bread, hot chocolate, fizzy drinks, capsicum, unpeeled cucumber and raw onion; and remove pizza from the takeaway menu. I suggested starting each day with a small bowl of seed mix for breakfast (see Appendix 3) moistened with a little apple or pear juice, or soy milk. Lunch could be either a sourdough rye **toasted** salad sandwich (bread is easier to digest when toasted) – no unpeeled cucumber – a tuna or salmon salad or an omelet. Dinner should be protein; that is, either chicken, fish, eggs or legumes (cooked with a bay leaf or a little seaweed) plus steamed or well-cooked stir-fried vegetables. Remember, no onions or capsicum, and any cruciferous vegetables should be very well cooked. (Although nutritionally speaking it is best not to overcook vegetables, in cases of poor digestion well cooked is the best option.) Brown rice, buckwheat or corn pasta could be included, if desired.

I discouraged takeaway meals for the time being. In fact, in the time Clare spent driving to a cafe or restaurant, then choosing, ordering and waiting for her takeaway meal, she could have gone home and steamed a delicious selection of vegetables to accompany either a can of salmon, scrambled eggs or some stir-fried tofu. If the cupboard at home was bare, then a quick stop at the local grocer for these ingredients would still be good time and meal management.

To encourage hydrochloric acid (HCl) production I asked Clare to sip a small glass of water with one teaspoon

of apple cider vinegar with her main meal. When this was
not possible, I gave Clare some potassium chloride tablets
to chew with the meal to stimulate HCl production. And,
of course, eating slowly in a relaxed manner was firmly
recommended. To relax the gut musculature I prescribed a
heavy-duty magnesium supplement to be taken before bed,
and herbal medicine to gently stimulate liver and gallbladder
function. Finally, Clare would keep a diet diary for a week,
making a particular note of any food-related digestive
discomfort.

Two weeks later Clare returned for her follow-up visit.
I am pleased to report there was marked improvement in her
bowel function and a 50 per cent reduction in her bloatedness.
After going through her revised eating regime with the
assistance of her diet diary, I was, however, suspicious that
Clare had some serious food allergies. There was a fairly
consistent pattern of bloating after breakfast, despite the new
healthy seed-mix routine (to which Clare added either oat or
barley bran), and there was also the occasional slight nausea
or bowel discomfort after an omelet-based lunch. In the initial
consultation I had checked whether there was a family history
of coeliac disease – which there was not – but I suspected
a possible gluten sensitivity, nonetheless. Clare agreed to a
food-allergy test and the results sent by the lab one week later
were illuminating. Clare had mild food allergies to barley, oat,
rye, wheat and millet. That is, all the gluten-containing grains
as well as millet. She also returned strong positive results for

allergies to cow's milk, pineapple, coffee and cola nut – the usual suspects. Egg white registered as a mild allergy, the same rating as the grains (this explained her reaction to omelet). We adjusted Clare's seed mix to a rice bran-based option rather than an oat-based one, replaced cow's milk yoghurt with sheep's milk or soy yoghurt, and removed all egg-based meals. Coffee was not a problem as Clare was not a coffee drinker, and cola nut no longer featured in her diet as she had already deleted the occasional Coke, as well as all other carbonated drinks. (Cola nut is an extremely common allergen found in cola-based drinks, such as Coke, as well as a range of lollies. See Chapter 9, Adverse food reactions: Allergies, sensitivities and intolerances.)

As the gluten-containing grains featured strongly in Clare's food-allergy test, I arranged for her to have a blood test for coeliac disease. Fortunately this proved negative, and after a three month total food-allergy exclusion diet we were able to safely reintroduce some of these troublesome grains. After this period of avoidance, any remaining sensitivity would be immediately and clearly noticed. However, a lifetime of eating foods that she was allergic to had damaged the mucosal lining of her small intestine. So, while on the total food-allergy exclusion diet, it was an opportune time to get in there and undertake some major repair work. I prescribed a glutamine-based supplement, to be taken twice a day before meals.

Within four weeks, after following the food-allergy exclusion diet in conjunction with the suggested anti-bloat measures, Clare was almost completely pain-free. This was the first time in over a decade she could remember not being bloated, and she was also having a daily bowel motion. Her energy levels had also improved – not surprisingly because gut pain is really and truly tiring. It takes a lot of our body's energy to respond to inflammation, and even mild constipation can make us feel sluggish and lethargic.

After Clare had been on the food-allergy exclusion diet for three months, we reintroduced the problematic grains and discovered that while barley, oat and millet were now well tolerated, wheat and rye still caused discomfort. Eggs in moderation no longer caused any nausea, but cow's milk invariably resulted in bloating and gut discomfort. Clare did not particularly like milk, so elimination was not a hardship. In fact, she discovered a passion for sheep's milk yoghurt and found a soy milk she liked, which, in conjunction with green leafy vegetables and almonds, ensured adequate calcium intake.

The herbal medicine was deleted after five months, and Clare continued to have complete and daily bowel motions. The herbs had restored optimum liver function, which could be maintained with a healthy diet. Clare's bloating episodes now occur only when she eats while anxious, or when she doesn't give herself sufficient time in the morning to chew her breakfast well **and** allow time for a bowel motion.

Gut flora imbalance

I did not need to investigate Clare's bowel flora as she did not have a history of antibiotic use, use the oral contraceptive pill (OCP), consume excessive sugar or alcohol or have a history of recurrent thrush. However, for many of my clients who have major bloating issues, an imbalance of gut flora is nearly always a significant factor. In the next chapter we examine the delicate relationship between gut microflora and bloating so we can easily identify it in a line up of 'pro-bloat' villains.

6

GUT FLORA:
GETTING THE BALANCE RIGHT

What is this microfloric world living so precariously in our gut, and what exactly does it do?

Our colon contains a plethora of 'friendly' intestinal bacteria – referred to as gut flora. In fact, approximately 5000 species of bacteria exist in the human body, and a healthy adult can carry as many as ten quadrillion individual bacteria in the gastrointestinal tract (GIT) alone! It is estimated that bacteria account for 30–50 per cent of the solid content of the human colon. Findings from the first large-scale study of the human colon genome, recently published in *Science,* claim that the human gut is as busy with microbes as the soils and the seas.

Some beneficial bacteria are implanted at birth – the birth canal is a rich source of the *Lactobacillus* species, and breast milk stimulates colonisation of bifidobacteria and lactobacilli in the newborn's gut – and the rest is acquired during later stages of life. These friendly bacteria strains usually inhabit the GIT, although they can be found in other cozy niches; acidophilus normally resides in the small intestine, and bifidus in the large intestine, or bowel. They do, however, cross bowel boundaries and can on occasion be found socialising in each other's homes. Our total wellbeing, not just our gastrointestinal health, depends on the maintenance of a balanced internal ecosystem. It is a fragile co-existence, easily disrupted by a number of factors. Let's establish what exactly our bowel flora does for us. They are, in twenty-first-century talk, multi-taskers, and are responsible for the:

- digestion and absorption of nutrients
- inhibition of pathogenic bacteria
- synthesis of B-group vitamins
- enhancement of the GIT's motility
- metabolism of plant compounds
- stimulation of the immune system
- production of short-chain fatty acids (SCFAs).

Maintaining a healthy, balanced gut flora depends on the foods we eat, the drugs we take and the state of our mind. The oral contraceptive pill (OCP), antibiotics, alcohol, excessive sugar and stress can dramatically alter the delicate microflora balance of our large and small intestines resulting in a multitude of gut-related symptoms, of which bloating is one. Stress increases the amount of aerobic bacteria, such as *Escherichia coli*, and decreases the amount of anaerobic bacteria, such as *Lactobacilli* and *Bifidobacteria*

(*Bifidobacteria* is particularly sensitive to stress). So, if you have recently completed a course of antibiotics or have used them on and off over the years, are taking the OCP, drink alcohol regularly, or snack on lollies or chocolate, then you need to consider the state of your friendly bacteria. Chances are that the bloating, diarrhoea, escalating food intolerances, constipation, halitosis (bad breath) or poor digestion you may be experiencing are due to a short supply on the micro-flora front.

Treatment of an imbalance of gut flora

There are two ways to address an imbalance or deficiency of friendly bacteria in the gut. One is to help manufacture beneficial bacteria by providing the fuel through appropriate dietary choices: *prebiotics*; the other is to introduce beneficial strains of bacteria with supplements: *probiotics*.

PREBIOTICS

Prebiotics are non-digestible carbohydrates that stimulate the growth of friendly bacteria in the colon. These carbohydrates are fermented in the colon into short-chain fatty acids (SCFAs) which provide the fuel to feed beneficial bacteria and assist in the repair of the gut wall. There are two main types of prebiotics: arabinogalactans and fructo-oligosaccharides.

The prebiotic arabinogalactans increases the populations of lactobacillus and bifidus (the healthy bacteria strains), and reduces the levels of toxic ammonia and the amount of pathogenic bacteria, such as *Escherichia coli*, present in our GIT. This prebiotic is generally derived for supplementation purposes from the Western larch tree, but it is also found in carrots, radishes, black beans, pear and maize.

Fructo-oligosaccharides (FOS) are a type of prebiotic some readers may be familiar with (psyllium, for example, is a FOS). They are known for their positive effect on the growth of healthy bacteria; however, I generally do not recommend this form of prebiotic therapy in cases of abdominal distension because we are unable to break down FOSs into simple sugars that can be absorbed by the intestine. As a result, they pass into the colon where they are digested, producing a large amount of carbon dioxide and other gases. Definitely not recommended for overcoming bloat. Other foods that contain FOSs include rye, oats, chicory, bananas, leeks, tomatoes, asparagus and onions.

Foods that contain inulin, a polysaccharide, such as Jerusalem artichokes and garlic are a good source of fuel for making colonies of friendly bacteria.

PROBIOTIC FOODS

Probiotics are beneficial micro-organisms that when ingested have a positive affect on the health of our intestinal flora. Sources include naturally fermented foods as well as, of course, a diverse range of supplements.

Naturally fermented foods could be called the original probiotic. Yoghurt, a fermented dairy product, is a well-known source of probiotics, but tempeh (see Appendix 5 for a truly delicious tempeh recipe), sauerkraut and sour-dough bread are also excellent sources.

In fact, *Lactobacillus casei*, the strain found in fermented dairy products, is resistant to antibiotics (which can detrimentally affect the balance of our gut flora), and consequently helps prevent diarrhoea following a course of antibiotics, particularly in children. What's more, this friendly strain of bacteria improves digestion and assimilation of dairy-based foods, which accounts for the fact that many people who cannot digest dairy are able to consume yoghurt without any difficulties. (Those who have a lactase deficiency are generally able to eat yoghurt as the bacterial process converts much of the lactose into lactic acid.) *L. casei* also helps break down the largely indigestible compounds present in soy. Both *Lactobacillus plantarum* and *Lactobacillus casei* are found in tempeh, sauerkraut and sourdough breads.

A note on yoghurt

Choosing the right yoghurt can be a challenge. The number of (inappropriate) options is a minefield, and it's easy to slip up and make a mistake. Full fat, low fat, no fat, low GI, organic, biodynamic, fruit, vanilla, Greek style, sheep's, goat's, cow's, soy! However, there are only two vital points to be mindful of: your yoghurt *must* contain several strains of friendly bacteria, such as *Lactobacillus acidophilus*, *Lactobacillus bulgaricus* or *Lactobacillus casei*; and it *must not* contain sugar. Sugar destroys our friendly bacteria. Not much point putting it in, only to destroy it in the same mouthful!

I would recommend, wherever possible, plain organic or biodynamic, low-fat yoghurt made with cow's, sheep's or goat's milk. If you can find soy yoghurt without a skerrick of sugar (not easy), then that too would be a good option. And vary your dairy sources: one week cow's, next week sheep's, because each type of milk contains a different proportion of protein, fat and water, and the fat globule size varies, making some milk far easier to digest than others. (See Appendix 6 for a guide to making your own yoghurt.)

PROBIOTIC SUPPLEMENTS

Generally speaking, there are two main species of bacteria found in the supplements normally prescribed: *Lactobacillus* and *Bifidobacterium*. Most bacteria have multiple actions and for optimum efficacy are generally prescribed in combination. Indeed, probiotic supplements that contain different species of beneficial bacteria most closely resemble the natural composition of our intestinal flora. The following is a basic description of the multiple strains of probiotics and their many functions.

Lactobacillus

The main strains of *Lactobacillus* are:

- *Lactobacillus acidophilus* is one of the most important inhabitants in the small intestine. It also exists in the lining of the vagina where it controls vaginal infections such as *Candida albicans*. It produces the enzyme lactase that helps in the management of lactose intolerance and inhibits the growth of pathogenic bacteria in the bowel, such as *Staphylococcus aureus*, *Salmonella typhimurium*, *Escherichia coli* and *Clostridium perfringens*. *L. acidophilus* may help reduce the risk of food sensitivities, prevents and reduces diarrhoea and vomiting, and alleviates bloating.

- *Lactobacillus plantarum 299v* increases the production of anti-inflammatory proteins in the mucosal immune system of our intestines (the centre of our immune system is in the GIT). This in turn reduces inflammation, making it the ideal probiotic for the treatment of inflammatory bowel disorders, such as Crohn's disease and ulcerative colitis. Its ability to improve gut flora populations and reduce the adhesion of pathogenic bacteria means it is a superb supplement to use following abdominal surgery. *L. plantarum* also modifies the 'anti-nutrients', substances that interfere with the absorption of nutrients in some foods, especially from whole grains and soy beans, allowing optimum nutrient uptake. Supplementation with *L. plantarum 299v* alleviates pain, regulates bowel habits and decreases flatulence in irritable bowel syndrome (IBS).

- *Lactobacillus rhamnosus* strengthens the gut wall's resistance to infection, and alleviates intestinal inflammation in infants suffering from atopic dermatitis or food allergy by improving the breast milk's immunoprotection potential. It also decreases hypersensivity to milk, prevents antibiotic-associated diarrhoea and is beneficial to sufferers of Crohn's disease.

- *Lactobacillus salivarius* is beneficial in the treatment of inflammatory bowel disease, and inhibits *Staphylococcus aureus* (golden staph).

- *Lactobacillus casei* improves the digestion and assimilation of dairy products and is resistant to antibiotics.

Bifidobacterium

Bifidobacteria comprise approximately 90 per cent of the beneficial bacteria of the large intestine, and, in general, enhance the function of the digestive system. They increase defecation frequency, faecal organic-acid content and water content, improve the faecal consistency and alleviate bloating. They also promote the synthesis in the intestinal tract of several B vitamins, including biotin and folic acid. *Bifidobacteria* are capable of reducing many pathogens and are effective in treating acute diarrhoea and rotavirus infection.

The main strains of *Bifidobacterium* are:

- *Bifidobacterium bifidum* inhibits many pathogens, including *Clostridium*, *Escherichia coli*, *Enterococccus*, *Helicobacter pylori* and *Staphylococcus*.
- *Bifidobacterium breve* is specifically located in the large intestine. It inhibits pathogens, such as *Escherichia coli*, *Enterococccus*, *Gardnerella vaginalis* and *Pseudomonas*.
- *Bifidobacterium longum* improves faecal consistency and visual characteristics, enhances the gut's immune defences and inhibits many pathogens, such as *Enterobacteriaceae*, *Clostridium* and *Escherichia coli*.

How to produce our own bifidobacteria

As mentioned, some foods act as prebiotics, encouraging the proliferation of beneficial bacteria. However, these indigestible prebiotics (oligosaccharides), when broken down by the gas-producing bacteria in the gut, can cause flatulence.

In 1994 it was discovered that the bacteria traditionally used as a starter in the manufacture of Swiss cheese,

Propionibacterium freudenreichii, encourages the growth of certain strains of *Bifidobacteria*. This rather unpronounceable, newly discovered bacterium increases levels of *B. longum, B. bifidum, B. adolentis* and *B. breve*. Indeed it is able to increase bifidobacterial levels in the body by up to 3000 per cent! In the process, it produces large amounts of vitamin B12, folic acid and anti-oxidants. Other worthy traits of *P. freudenreichii* are its ability to inhibit moulds, yeast (such as *Candida albicans*), bacteria and viruses; and to reduce the risk of liver cancer by blocking the absorption of fungal toxin (aflatoxin), which is a powerful liver carcinogen. Also in its favour is its hardiness. Unlike many strains of beneficial bacteria, it is heat stable over a wide pH range, resistant to many enzymes, especially to acid, thereby able to reach the intestine relatively intact and active.

Other probiotic strains

- *Streptococcus thermophilus* is a beneficial strain of the *Streptococcus* bacteria that rapidly acidifies the intestinal environment, creating a milieu favourable to lactobacillus. It quells digestive inflammation, enhances the immune system, reduces symptoms in allergic patients and prevents antibiotic-induced diarrhoea. It is widely used in the manufacture of cheese and yoghurt.
- *Saccharomyces boulardii* is a beneficial strain of

yeast, first discovered in the skin of the lychee fruit. In France it is popularly called the 'yeast against yeast' because, as it becomes established, it crowds out unfriendly strains of yeast, such as candida. I have had some stunning results using it to treat resistant cases of gastrointestinal and vaginal candida infections. However, those with a true yeast allergy (that is, when ingestion results in anaphylactic shock) must avoid *S. boulardii*.

In the gut *S. boulardii* produces lactic acid, some B vitamins, decreases gut permeability, reduces harmful bacteria and treats infectious diarrhoea and antibiotic diarrhoea. It is also effective in the treatment of digestive discomfort associated with food sensitivities by improving the body's metabolism of carbohydrates. It does this by increasing the activity of our digestive enzymes: sucrase, maltase and lactase.

Getting the most from your probiotic

The successful arrival of a probotic supplement into our small and large intestine is not an easy task. In fact, tests show that only 30–67 per cent of *Bifidobacteria* supplementation arrives safely in the bowel. It is a minefield down there. The probiotic must survive the onslaught of gastrointestinal secretions, such as hydrochloric acid (HCl), bile salts and pancreatic enzymes. How can we maximise their survival rate? The following suggestions will help you get the most from probiotic supplements:

- Take your supplement on an empty stomach, and preferably in a capsule with an 'enteric' coating to protect it against the acidic stomach and intestinal secretions. If the bacterial strains are acid-resistant, the coating is not so important (*L. acidophilus*, *L. plantarum*, *L. casei*, *L. rhamnosus* and *B. longum* are extremely acid-resistant).

- Regular supplementation (*not* the stop-start 'I forgot to take my supplement' approach) will maximise the growth of friendly bacteria. And to be most effective your supplement must contain at least 25 billion organisms. (The majority of probiotic supplements range from 12–25 billion organisms.)

- Provide an intestinal environment conducive to the adherence and growth of friendly bacteria by including sufficient fibre, such as oat bran, whole grains, fruit and vegetables with skins, as well as oily fish and flaxseed oil in your diet.

- Ensure the probiotic supplement is of human origin, which is more likely to survive and replicate than those from the intestinal environment of a pig or a cow. Multi-strain probiotic supplements offer the most complete spectrum of friendly bacteria. Probiotics containing a mix of human (e.g. *L. acidophilus*), dairy (e.g. *Streptococcus thermophilus*) and vegetal (e.g. *L. plantarum*) sources appear to have a complementary synergistic action.

- Check which binder is used in the probiotic supplement and choose one that does not contain a potentially allergenic additive. For instance, some probiotic capsules and powders are filled with maltodextrin – a type of starch derived from either wheat or corn that will, naturally, cause a reaction in wheat- or corn-sensitive people.

- Supplement with a probiotic while taking antibiotics, but ensure it is a multi-strain formula *not* a single strain. Recent research suggests that some probiotic strains are resistant to certain antibiotics. Results published in *Current Microbiology* in 2005 indicated that strains of *Lactobacillus* and *Bifidobacterium* (*L. acidophilus, L. rhamnosus, L. brevis* and *B. longum*) were resistant to the antibiotics erythromycin and clindamycin. Other laboratory tests showed that a number of strains of *Lactobacillus* and *Bifidobacterium* showed resistance to a further 13 commonly prescribed antibiotics (see Appendix 7 for the complete list of antibiotics).

- Refrigerate your probiotic supplement at 4–6 °C to ensure the bacteria retains maximum quality to the end of its shelf-life. However, short-term periods of up to three days outside refrigerated conditions shouldn't affect your supplement unduly as long as it remains sealed and away from direct sunlight.

7

CONSTIPATION:
WHAT'S THE HOLD UP?

'For love of God to take some laxative;
Upon my soul that's the advice to give
For melancholy choler; let me urge
You free yourself from vapours with a purge.'
— *Canterbury Tales,* CHAUCER
(Pertetole to Chanticleer . . . Fortunately, Chanticleer rejected Pertetoles' advice!)

A question I ask every client, no matter what the reason they have come to see me, is: 'Do you have a daily bowel motion?' Some clients answer rather too quickly, giving a brief, embarrassed nod or an almost inaudible 'No, not daily', wishing to move on to a different subject as soon as possible. Others are unsure, needing time to consider their bowel frequency, as they have not taken much notice of it in the past. A small minority take to the subject matter with enthusiasm, detailing the time, consistency, variation, regularity, colour and form. I encourage everyone to take an active interest in this matter. It is of vital importance. A daily, satisfactory bowel motion is *crucial* to good health.

What is 'normal'?

A daily, complete, easy-to-expel bowel motion is desirable and achievable. Faeces should be full, rounded, soft, brown to light brown in colour and easily broken up when the toilet is flushed. Ideally, we should have a bowel movement at the same time each morning; probably after breakfast. We can train our bodies to be regular (tips to follow on page 72) as bowel habits are just that – habits which can be acquired and maintained. Transit time in the gastrointestinal tract (GIT) is, on average, about 16–24 hours; although, it can take some people up to 72 hours to complete this vital function.

Constipation refers to infrequent or difficult defecation, and is defined as either: fewer than three bowel movements per week, with the total volume of stools passed each day less than 35 g (250 g is ideal – try to imagine this weight, no need to be exact!), or there is difficulty, pain or incomplete passing of stools.

Bowel-transit-time test

There is a simple test to assess your bowel-transit time that can be performed in the privacy of your own home. Inexpensive, pain-free and even enjoyable! Simply lunch on corn or include some roughly chopped beetroot in your salad at midday and watch for its arrival in the toilet bowl. The remnants should appear some time between 6.00 and 9.00 am the following day. Any later than this indicates a seriously sluggish bowel and needs to be investigated. But first check your daily fibre and water intake, which should be approximately 50 g and 2 L, respectively. If necessary, adjust your intake and retest (see Appendix 8, Fibre figures).

The mechanics of a bowel motion

If we reflect back on Chapter 2, when we took our trip through the GIT, you may remember that the major role of the large intestine is the absorption of water and the fermentation of unabsorbed and undigested carbohydrates. The contents of our large intestine are moved along by a series of peristaltic movements, ultimately arriving at the rectum. The contents stretch the walls of the rectum forcing the anal sphincter to relax, which creates the urge to have a bowel motion (known as the defecation or rectal reflex). Adults, unlike infants, have control of the external anal sphincter, meaning we can constrict the sphincter and postpone defecation. The faeces, consequently, backup into the sigmoid colon until the next wave of peristalsis again stimulates the rectum, creating the need to defecate. If we repeatedly ignore this urge to use our bowels, the rectum eventually stops signalling when defecation is needed and we end up with an uncomfortable case of chronic constipation.

Yes, I know, no one except naturopaths enjoy talking about their bowels, but sometimes we just have to bite the bullet and (briefly) examine the ins and outs of our large intestine.

Tips for good bowel habits

- Don't ignore that urge! As soon as you feel the need to go to the toilet, attend to it straight away. This will encourage regular bowel habits and then your answer to my question: 'Do you have a daily bowel motion?' will be 'Like clockwork. The same time every day!' Music to my ears.

- Diet and exercise are the keys to a regular bowel habit. We need to consume 30–50 g of fibre and about 2 L of water a day (depending on physical activity, weight and climate) to have a complete and satisfying daily bowel motion. Exercise also stimulates peristalsis and tones the muscles of the abdomen and large intestine. Brisk walking is perfect.

- Your position on the toilet seat counts! (Don't squirm, this will only take a minute to explain and may resolve a lot of unnecessary time and *effort* in the bathroom.) Squatting is truly the best position – not easy with Western-style toilets. However, here is a dignified version you can try: sit on the toilet seat and place your feet on top of a small stool (probably not a good choice of word in this context) or a stack of magazines, thus raising your knees. This will slightly change the angle of your anal passage, relaxing the anal sphincters and triggering the urge to empty your bowel.

- Do not rush your daily routine. Establish a regular pattern of going to the toilet at the same time each day, allow yourself sufficient time and try to relax. Also, drink a glass of warm water and lemon juice on rising. This is a gentle liver stimulant and will stimulate a bowel movement.

Symptoms of constipation

The American humorist Josh Billings wrote: 'I have finally come to the conclusion that a good reliable set of bowels is worth more to a man than any quantity of brains.' While a little overzealous in his appreciation of regularity, Mr Billings has a point.

The large intestine, or colon, is a temporary storage tank for waste matter. This waste material needs to be removed within 16 to 24 hours, otherwise the harmful toxins that form after this period may cause a number of serious conditions, such as migraine (you may be familiar with the expression 'toxic migraine'), and even appendicitis and diverticulitis.

Chronic constipation can make our lives very uncomfortable, resulting in a range of symptoms including:

- bad breath (halitosis)
- body odour
- acne
- headaches
- abdominal distension and pain
- varicose veins
- indigestion
- fatigue
- hernias
- haemorrhoids
- weight gain
- poor sleep.

Most symptoms are totally reversible, once optimal bowel function has been achieved.

Causes of constipation

Most common causes of constipation are:

- poor bowel habits
- lack of dietary fibre
- insufficient fluids
- excessive intake of certain fibre, such as wheat bran, or psyllium taken without sufficient water
- high-protein/low-carb diets
- lack of muscle tone

- lack of exercise
- stress and anxiety
- overuse of laxatives and enemas
- pharmaceutical drugs; such as pain killers and anti-depressants
- inorganic iron supplements
- pregnancy.

A less common cause is rebound constipation, which can occur following the use of anti-diarrhoea drugs or the consumption of charcoal tablets (see Chapter 5, Banish the bloat). More serious factors to consider include: metabolic and endocrine abnormalities (such as hypothyroidism, hypercalcaemia, hypokalaemia and uraemia); structural, muscular and neurogenic abnormalities of the colon or spine; hernias, prolapses, diverticular disease and bowel cancer. These serious conditions require medical diagnosis.

Treatment of constipation

The following regime can be followed by anyone suffering from chronic constipation. However, first ensure that there are no structural abnormalities, bowel disease or any other more serious causes.

DIET AND LIFESTYLE

- Start the day with a glass of warm water and lemon juice.

- Consume at least 50 g of dietary fibre every day.
- Drink a minimum of 1½–2 L of water every day.
- Include bitter greens in your daily diet.
- Use or adapt the seed-mix recipe as your breakfast ritual.
- Add 5 ml flaxseed oil to food twice a day.
- Do not eat red meat, dairy*, especially yellow cheese (plain, 'live' yoghurt is fine), and white carbohydrates (think white rice, bread, pasta, cakes).
- If constipation is entrenched, drink 30 ml aloe vera juice twice a day on an empty stomach, maintain this for two weeks only.
- Elevate feet while on the toilet seat or squat.
- Massage your abdomen while lying in bed in the morning (see page 78).
- Leave enough time in the morning to have a bowel motion.
- Chew each mouthful well before swallowing.
- Exercise regularly, such as brisk walking, swimming and Pilates.
- Practise deep-diaphragmatic breathing, often incorporated in yoga (this can stimulate peristalsis by correcting abdominal pressure).
- Maintain a sense of humour, which can be difficult I know, but belly laughter is especially stimulating – being likened to internal jogging!

*Note: a European study, cited in the Journal of Pediatrics, *found that three out of four children with constipation had a form of intestinal immune reaction – lymphonodular hyperplasia – which is associated with cow's milk allergy. After analysing the results,* The Australian Medical Observer *recommended that small children with severe chronic constipation should trial a milk-free diet.*

SUPPLEMENTS

- magnesium: 800 mg a day, taken in a divided dose; e.g. 200 mg at breakfast and at dinner, and 400 mg before bed. Use either magnesium amino acid chelate or a combination of magnesium orotate and magnesium aspartate.
- vitamin B complex (check it includes at least 50 mg of most of the B vitamins)
- probiotics, particularly *Bifidobacterium lactis*, taken on an empty stomach, twice a day.

HERBS

Herbal medicine should especially include liver and gall-bladder herbs, such as fringe tree, globe artichoke, St Mary's thistle and dandelion root (see your naturopath or herbalist). If there is a great deal of abdominal tension, calming and relaxing herbs such as cramp bark, lemon balm, verbena and lime blossom should be prescribed.

INTESTINAL MASSAGE

I recommend massaging your abdomen first thing in the morning while lying in bed. Use either your fist or a pair of rolled up socks.

In a clockwise direction, starting at the lower-right corner of your abdomen (imagine where your appendix is – or was – located), gently massage in a circular motion: up the right-hand side of your abdomen, along and under the rib cage and then down the left-hand side, to the lower-left pelvic region. Breathe gently. Repeat three times.

This stimulates peristalsis, gently pushing things along, so to speak.

A DISCOURAGING WORD ON LAXATIVES AND COLONIC IRRIGATION

A warning: be very careful in your use of laxatives as they can be habit-forming. Long-term use, which is in fact abuse, of laxatives results in irreversible constipation. Habitual use of laxatives damages the nerve cells in the wall of the colon, decreasing the force of contractions. The bowel loses its muscle tone and its peristaltic ability, making the normal urge to defecate a difficult and painful experience. Harsher and harsher laxatives must be used to have an effect, creating a vicious cycle of constipation and laxative dependency.

I have seen too many colonoscopy reports that state the colon was unable to be examined clearly due to the blackening of the mucous membranes caused by the long-term use of senna-containing laxatives. Just because it is herbal doesn't mean it is safe. There are less stimulating herbs available that have a similar effect without the harshness of senna (aloe vera, for example). It should be noted, nonetheless, that all laxative herbs containing anthraquinone glycosides, such as aloe vera, cascara, yellow dock and senna, are not recommended in cases of abdominal pain of unknown origin and acute inflammatory diseases, such as Crohn's disease and ulcerative colitis, and pregnancy.

Laxatives commonly known as 'stool softeners', such as mineral oil and docusate sodium, may cause liver damage, and if inhaled can harm the delicate tissue of the lungs. They also interfere with the absorption of fat-soluble vitamins. Likewise, laxatives such as epsom salts and milk of magnesia, which act as osmotic agents (that is, they contain salts or carbonates that promote the secretion of water into the colon), also wash out minerals from the body.

The only times a herbal laxative is acceptable is when:

- there has been a long history of constipation and harsh methods are required, as a one-off, to clear the bowel in order to begin corrective treatment
- there is acute, life-threatening constipation; for example, due to a twisted bowel
- there has been some form of spinal injury, resulting in damage or destruction to the nerves that regulate bowel movement

- your bowel has suffered through a long plane
  journey. A combination of stodgy in-flight
  food and a situation not conducive to emptying
  the bowel may require a laxative, as a one-off
  measure.

Now for colonic irrigations. *Never* have a colonic irrigation. This unnecessary procedure refers to the passing of a rubber tube through the rectum for a distance up to 50–57 cm. Warm water, sometimes up to 75 L or more, is pumped in and out through the tube, a few litres at a time, to wash out the contents of the large intestine. Some practioners add herbs, coffee, wheat-grass extract and other substances to the enema solution. As you can imagine this procedure is rather uncomfortable, not to mention expensive, and it has considerable potential for harm.

The presence of a tube inserted into the bowel can cause cramping and pain, and if the equipment is not sterilised properly between treatments germs from one person's large intestine can be transmitted to another's. The mere thought of this type of cross-infection should be enough to dissuade anyone from having a colonic. Other dangers that have been reported include: bowel perforation, a possible and deadly consequence of poorly performed colonic irrigations, heart failure from excessive fluid absorbed into the bloodstream, fluid retention, altered pH balance and muscle cramps. Clients who have undergone a colonic irrigation procedure frequently report subsequent cases of constipation and thrush. If there is anything to 'clean out' this can safely be achieved by bulking laxatives, abdominal massage and gentle herbal medicine.

The so-called decaying faecal matter wondrously displayed in colonic-irrigation advertisements, conveniently shaped like your large intestine, is often the mucous lining – the *protective* mucous lining – of your hard-working large intestine. *Not* to be removed under any circumstances. The friendly bowel flora that live in your bowel, trying hard to maintain a healthy bowel environment, are often ripped out in the colonic irrigation frenzy. Hence the occurrence of vaginal thrush or *Candida* following time spent on the incline board at your local colonic irrigation centre.

In my years in practice, I have treated far too many clients suffering the serious consequences of their addiction to colonic irrigation.

....

Mary came to see me about a skin problem – she was 38 years old and still got regular outbreaks of acne – but it soon became apparent that she also had a bowel problem. And the two conditions were definitely connected.

When I asked Mary about her bowel function she said: 'Oh, I've never been regular, I've always had a sluggish bowel, and it doesn't seem to matter how much fibre I eat. I'm lucky to go twice a week. My mother's the same, must be a family trait.' Clearly not good. The two bowel motions she was able to obtain each week were a struggle, often resembling rabbit pellets and they always felt incomplete. Mary had in fact been hospitalised twice in the past with bowel impaction, which is unfortunate but at least it meant she had undergone a series of thorough investigations, including a colonoscopy, endoscopy and full blood test. Thankfully, all had come back normal, so we could rule out any structural abnormalities in the bowel, or serious gallbladder or liver disease. She had not, however, been asked a single question about her diet, although her doctor had once recommended she eat more bran.

An iris analysis revealed a fairly toxic system, physiological stress in the gut region and a slightly acid stomach zone. Mary also had numerous 'nerve arcs' in the outer regions of her iris, indicating she had been or was currently experiencing considerable stress. In addition, a tongue examination revealed a thick white coating meaning poor digestion and a possible imbalance of gut flora.

Mary's diet was similarly revealing. Despite her genuine belief that she had 'a healthy diet', there was clearly not enough fibre. Breakfast was frequently skipped altogether, or else it was a couple of pieces of fruit or a fruit smoothie. (Please do not drink your breakfast; there can never be enough fibre in a liquid meal. This is definitely one of my pet hates and I struggle to resist the urge to tut-tut when a client tells

me they have a smoothie for breakfast 'because it is quick'.)
She had raisin toast or a 'healthy' muffin at mid morning
and lunch was either a chicken or cheese and salad sandwich,
usually on rye bread; or a couple of nori rolls. Mid-afternoon
snack was normally a dry biscuit and cheese or a low-fat
yoghurt. Dinner was a salad with either steak, chops or
chicken; or pasta with a tomato-based sauce.

Mary's daily fibre count would be lucky to total 25 g (see
Appendix 8, Fibre figures), 50 per cent short of the amount
required to ensure a quick-and-easy daily bowel movement.
This is a common problem for those who skip breakfast, as
most of our dietary fibre is obtained through eating grains.
A startling example is the fact that half-a-cup of processed
bran cereal provides 10 g fibre compared to three cups cooked
broccoli or six nectarines. A simple bowl of a high-fibre
homemade seed mix has resolved many a case of chronic
constipation.

Mary drank about six glasses of water on a good day,
but this frequently dropped to two glasses a day, especially
on days when she was 'on the road'. This is fairly common
amongst my clients with jobs that involve a lot of time in the
car. Anxiety about needing to stop and find a toilet prevents
many people from achieving adequate hydration. But surely
a constipation-free life is worth the minor irritation of a few
stop-offs on the way?

In addition to Mary's two to six glasses of water each day,
she also drank three to four cups of tea with milk. The caffeine

in the tea is dehydrating – all the more reason to drink extra water – and the tannins were contributing to her constipation by having an astringent effect on the mucous membranes of the digestive tract. (As we shall see later, naturopaths and herbalists use tannin-rich herbs to treat diarrhoea as they bind the tissue of the gut and form a protective layer on the membranous tissue of our intestines. So, excessive tea drinking and constipation are not good bed, or should I say bowel fellows.) The milk was also potentially problematic – difficult to digest and constipating if drunk to excess. While many beverages, such as tea, coffee, sugary soft drinks and alcohol appear to quench thirst because they contain a high percentage of water, they are ultimately dehydrating; completely failing to meet our cell's requirements for water at the physiological level.

Although Mary loved her job, she was a senior sales rep for a high-profile European lingerie company, her long working day meant she was doing very little in the way of regular exercise (regular exercise + well-balanced diet = regular bowel). She tried to fit in a seven-kilometre walk around Melbourne's Botanic Gardens on the weekends, but this was clearly not enough. She had, to her credit, enrolled in Pilates lessons at the local gym, but was often so exhausted in the evening that by the time she got home she didn't have the energy to go or had missed the class due to late client appointments.

Mary's skin problems were undoubtedly related to

a history of constipation. The endotoxins (internally derived toxins) from the undigested and unexpelled food molecules, normally eliminated via the bowels, re-enter circulation. This causes a system overload, resulting in a quasi expulsion of the toxic material through one of our other organs of elimination, in Mary's case her skin. We have four main organs responsible for the excretion of waste products and water: the bowels, the kidneys, the lungs and the skin. A dysfunction in the elimination capacity of any one of these organs will put an increased burden on one or all of the others. The skin is responsible for the excretion of approximately one-quarter of the body's waste products. Interesting and relevant to note that Mary was also experiencing a great deal of fluid retention. Her face was slightly puffy and her ankles swollen, largely due to the overload on her kidneys because of her poor bowel function and inadequate water consumption.

Clearly, the first place to start was with Mary's diet. Fibre and water needed immediate attention. Mary's first task in the morning was to drink a large glass of warm water and lemon juice, designed to give our liver a gentle, but stimulating shove; it is also very beneficial for our skin and complexion. Mary needed to consume at least 50 g fibre each day. I asked her to do a daily fibre count and provided a fibre chart so there could be no miscalculations! The fibre chart would help her choose the right types and amount of food she needed to consume to reach her daily requirement.

I gave Mary a 'strongly recommended' menu to follow as

a guide, as initially it can be a bit daunting to know where to start. It looked like this:

Breakfast: four tablespoons of seed mix, moistened with a handful of raisins soaked in water overnight (use the water as well), half a cup of good-quality yoghurt and a generous metric teaspoon of flaxseed oil.

Lunch: a sourdough multigrain salad sandwich (with the bread merely holding all the salad components together) of beetroot, carrot, alfalfa sprouts, lettuce, spinach, plus any other favourite vegetables; or a huge salad plus either salmon, egg, chickpeas, kidney beans or lentils.

Dinner: to include at least five, and preferably seven, different vegetables (green and orange) and a protein, which could be chicken, fish, egg, tofu or legumes, but no red meat. Brown rice, wholemeal pasta or a baked potato with its skin, could be added, if desired. Each evening meal to be accompanied by a salad of bitter greens, with a lemon and olive oil dressing (that is, **as well as** the vegetables).

Snacks: fresh fruit (no more than one banana) or a few dried figs, half a cup of yoghurt and berries or brown rice cakes and hummus. I asked Mary to keep a diet diary for one week, noting her bowel movements beside each day's dietary and fibre intake, and to fax it back to me prior to our next consultation. This would give me time to analyse her fibre intake and to ensure there were no nutritional gaps.

I gave Mary a herbal tonic for liver and gallbladder function, and a magnesium supplement – a fairly hefty dose – to relax the gut musculature; a good-quality probiotic to reinoculate the bowel with the appropriate friendly flora, to be taken twice a day before meals (this would have the added benefit of improving her skin); and a high-dose vitamin B complex to protect the nervous system, help in the manufacture of bowel flora and improve the skin.

In addition to the dietary changes and the supplement regime, I recommended getting up 45 minutes earlier each day so she would have plenty of time to actually have a bowel movement. Rushing around in the morning, nervously gulping breakfast down at the same time as getting dressed and feeding the cat, is not conducive to a satisfactory bowel motion. I suggested, as diplomatically as possible, that Mary place a few phone books under her feet while sitting on the toilet seat, in order to place her anatomy in a more favourable eliminative position.

We tried to find an exercise regime that would fit into Mary's busy lifestyle, and agreed upon a brisk walk three times a week, combined with either regular Pilates or yoga (both excellent work outs for the bowel, as is belly dancing). Regular exercise would also improve Mary's skin – the lymphatic system doesn't have an independent pump (unlike the circulatory system, which has the heart) and relies on our arm and leg muscles to move lymphatic fluid and remove toxins out of the body.

I am happy to report that within two weeks Mary was having a bowel movement every second day, without *struggling, and by six weeks we had achieved a daily, complete motion, without straining or stress. Mary's skin had also cleared up significantly, with only the occasional outbreak. At the end of three months, Mary could hardly believe the change in her total wellbeing: clear skin, constipation-free, no more puffiness and increased energy. At this point I decreased her herbs and carefully cut back the magnesium supplementation. Within six months the only supplement Mary was taking was a low-dose magnesium and a high-dose vitamin B complex.*

*Mary still needs to be very careful not to deviate too much from a high-fibre diet, and finds that when she is time-pressured or under considerable stress she will occasionally experience a missed bowel motion. When this happens, Mary increases her magnesium for a few days, and things normally correct themselves. (Readers of **Revive** may remember that when we are stressed we release cortisol which decreases the levels of magnesium in our cells; however, when we are under stress our requirements for magnesium actually increase.)*

8

DIARRHOEA:
AN EXPLOSIVE EXPLORATION

Jeremy's first words to me were: 'It doesn't seem to matter what I eat. For the past few years I've been having episodes of uncontrollable diarrhoea, at least twice a week. Sometimes it's just loose or runny, yet at other times it can be positively explosive. I find this especially embarrassing at work when I often have to dash from a meeting. And my co-workers now avoid the shared office toilets after I've used them. I'm at my wits end.'

Jeremy is not alone in this uncomfortable and embarrassing situation. Diarrhoea, while not quite as common as its distant cousin constipation, is a serious problem for a fair percentage of the population. And it can potentially be life-threatening, especially in young children. We will return to Jeremy's case later in the chapter, but first let's clarify this problem of diarrhoea.

What is diarrhoea?

The hallmarks of diarrhoea are: frequent, loose or watery

stools, which may be explosive and/or uncontrollable and are often accompanied by cramping, nausea or vomiting, fever or excessive thirst. Diarrhoea occurs when the faeces pass through the colon too quickly, not allowing enough time for the normal re-absorption of water. The stools remain liquidy, resulting in frequent bowel movements.

The gastrointestinal tract (GIT) is a very busy place, with nerves, micro-organisms and immune cells all working to maintain a healthy order. A minor upset to any of these three elements will disrupt this delicate balance, invariably resulting in diarrhoea.

Causes of diarrhoea

- infection, viral or bacterial
- food poisoning
- drinking contaminated water
- intestinal parasites
- inflammatory bowel disease, such as Crohn's disease and ulcerative colitis
- certain foods, such as unripe fruits, spoiled or rancid foods
- caffeine and alcohol
- food intolerances and sensitivities
- stress
- antibiotics
- gut flora imbalance
- bowel prolapse

- nutritional deficiency, especially zinc*
- diseases of the liver and pancreas

*Note: a zinc deficiency can cause diarrhoea by decreasing the effectiveness of our immune response to pathogenic bacteria, exacerbating a leaky gut wall and increasing the likelihood of a hypersensitivity to food and environmental allergens. Children are often low in zinc which can predispose them to diarrhoea.

Treatment of diarrhoea – general

Treatment will, of course, vary according to the cause. If, for example, diarrhoea is due to stress and anxiety, I would prescribe nervine herbs and vitamins and minerals that soothe the nervous system (such as B vitamins and calcium). If, however, diarrhoea is a result of intestinal infection, then anti-parasitic and anti-microbial herbs would be used in conjunction with specific dietary measures, such as the elimination of sugar and yeasts. The most vital factor is to accurately identify the cause. Once this has been confidently established, then relevant measures can be prescribed. Thankfully, there are some sound general principles that can be followed by those experiencing the occasional bout of diarrhoea. However, if the diarrhoea continues for longer than three days, or is accompanied by blood, fever or severe pain, see your health care practitioner immediately. Diarrhoea is potentially fatal.

DIET

Eliminate the following:

- stimulants, such as alcohol and foods containing caffeine
- fatty foods
- all known or suspected food allergies and sensitivities
- dairy (except yoghurt)
- fruit (except grated apple, baked apple or pear, or a firm banana).

Include the following:

- a very simple diet, such as rice and vegetables, soups, toast, porridge
- left-over liquid from cooked rice and vegetables, as a broth
- meadowsweet tea throughout the day (especially beneficial for children with diarrhoea and sore tummies), it has a gentle astringent effect, reduces fever and relieves pain. (See Appendix 9 for further insights into this delightful herbal friend.)
- a large mug of strong chamomile tea after dinner.

SUPPLEMENTS

- half a teaspoon *Lactobacillus acidophilus* twice a day before meals
- add two teaspoons of psyllium to a glass of water,

drink before breakfast and follow with a *large* glass of water

- mix one teaspoon of slippery elm bark powder into a paste, then add 200 ml of water, and drink before meals twice a day. This is especially helpful for those with acute Crohn's disease. The bark powder is very soothing to an inflamed and irritated digestive system.
- herbal medicine includes: meadowsweet, chamomile, oak bark, bayberry, marshmallow, cramp bark
- check for zinc deficiency and supplement with zinc sulphate if required. Add 2 ml liquid zinc to 200 ml water, drink with food twice a day, or more frequently if required.
- rehydrate with the electrolyte minerals: sodium, potassium, calcium and, especially, magnesium. Use a good-quality formula containing a specifically formulated ratio of electrolytes that parallel those found in muscle cells. *No* salt tablets, please! Alternatively, make up a batch of mineral-dense rehydration soup, see below, and drink several cups throughout the day.

Rehydration soup
   2 potatoes with the skin, well scrubbed
   2 carrots

1 small celeriac root
½ bunch parsley
½ bunch spinach
2 teaspoons grated fresh ginger root
Celtic salt to taste
½ cup organic white rice or basmati rice

Roughly chop vegetables and place in a large saucepan. Add just enough filtered water to cover, add the rice and bring to a gentle boil. Cover and simmer for half an hour. Leave to stand for 10 minutes, drink hot or cold.

INSTANT ANTI-DIARRHOEA REMEDY

In a small bowl place half a cup of good-quality yoghurt containing the probiotic strains of *Lactobacillus acidophilus*, *Lactobacillus rhamnosus*, *Bifidobacterium longum* or *Lactobacillus casei*. Mix with half a grated apple that has oxidised (once it has turned brown), add one heaped teaspoon of slippery elm bark powder and sprinkle generously with freshly ground cinnamon. Eat slowly in a relaxed manner, chewing well. Follow with a cup of meadowsweet tea, sipped at a leisurely pace.

Treatment of diarrhoea – specific

ANTIBIOTIC-ASSOCIATED DIARRHOEA

Very few of us will escape at least one course of antibiotics in our lifetime, and antibiotics, as we are only too aware, often cause what is known as rebound diarrhoea. This can be prevented, however, by taking a few simple measures. First, take a good-quality probiotic supplement at the same time as you commence the antibiotic therapy. It must contain *Lactobacillus rhamnosus*. This strain of probiotic has been proven to prevent antibiotic-associated diarrhoea. Take it (on an empty stomach) for the entire time you are on the antibiotic and continue for at least two weeks afterwards. Alternatively, eat half a cup of a yoghurt that contains this strain daily (check labels for probiotic strains). At the same time, take a vitamin B complex each morning to ensure you manufacture your own friendly bacteria. And a diet rich in fermented foods, such as yoghurt, sauerkraut and tempeh will also assist. Avoid all alcohol and sugar.

If you are prone to thrush following a course of antibiotics, then the best probiotic to use is *Saccharomyces boulardii*, as this will displace the unfriendly candida yeast and stimulate an appropriate immune response. Take it while you are on the antibiotics and continue for two to four days afterwards. (See page 64.)

PARASITIC DIARRHOEA

Parasitic diarrhoea can occur in a number of ways. Consider the following common scenarios: while travelling overseas you have caught a bad case of 'traveller's tummy' and your bowel has 'never been well since'; you regularly drink tank water (the blastocystis parasite is found in stored water); or perhaps you have been in close contact with an infected pet. It is essential to determine the causative pathogen, and the best method is to have a *thorough* stool analysis, which your naturopath can arrange. Some pathology labs not only identify the pathogen but also test drugs and herbs against the infecting organism and advise the most effective remedy to use (see Appendix 2, Complete digestive stool analysis (CDSA)). The priority in this case of diarrhoea is to kill the parasite and then re-inoculate the bowel with friendly bacteria.

Parasitic-related diarrhoea is often accompanied by bloating, gas, general malaise and sometimes intestinal pain. Our first task is to rid ourselves of the infecting agent – why play intestinal host to unwanted visitors? If you suspect a parasitic infection, then herbal medicine is the place to start. We have a truly wonderful array of anti-parasitic tonics in the plant kingdom to choose from. A combination of anti-microbial herbs, such as Chinese wormwood, cat's claw, black walnut and grapefruit seed should do the trick. These herbs are normally available in tablet form, so no nasty liquid herbs to swallow. I can hear a collective sigh of relief! As a herbalist, I am quite adept at taking even the most bitter of herbs with barely a grimace, but even I have to admit that the anti-parasitic herbs are very unappetising. In tablet form, however, they slip down without the slightest curling of the lip. They will need to be taken for anything between four and eight weeks, depending on the severity and extent of the infection and whether it is local (i.e. specific to the GIT) or systemic.

Following this course of herbs it is vital to reintroduce friendly bacteria into the gut. Remember, an imbalance of gut flora can alter the immune response of the intestinal mucous lining – that is, it could result in a leaky gut. And it is bad enough having an unwanted visitor in your gut, let alone your bloodstream or other organs. The best choice in a supplement is a combination of acidophilus and bifidus. The beauty of our probiotic friend is that not only will it restore a balanced flora to our GIT but it will also prevent and control the growth of pathogenic organisms.

STRESS-ASSOCIATED DIARRHOEA

Follow the general guidelines for treating diarrhoea but also address the underlying cause: a hypersensitive nervous system or an overly stretched one. It is most important to take a high-potency vitamin B complex, in addition to a combined calcium and magnesium supplement (start on 400 mg calcium hydroxyapatite or calcium citrate, and 200 mg magnesium orotate or citrate a day). These will exert a calming effect and decrease anxiety. In addition, herbal medicine is strongly recommended. Herbs such as oats seed, lemon balm, lime blossom, verbena, skullcap and chamomile are especially soothing for gut-related disorders. Your naturopath or herbalist can make up a blend to suit your individual constitution. A herbal tonic I have found particularly help-ful for stress-affected bowels is the following blend: oats 30 ml, cramp bark 20 ml, lime flowers 20 ml and chamomile 30 ml. Take 5 ml three times a day with meals.

This gentle herbal blend is calming and relaxing to the gut as well as restorative to a drained, strained nervous system. Take over a two-to-three-month period.

And don't let us forget Bach flowers! Bach flowers are homeopathic remedies that address the major moods of the psyche, such as fear, despair and over-sensitivity. The Bach Rescue Remedy, a combination of five individual Bach flower remedies, is the ultimate calming homeo-pathic tool. It may be taken as often as every ten minutes in extremely stressful circumstances, such as pre-exam or pre-public-presentation nervous bowels; or alternatively, it can be taken two to four times a day as a more general, behind-the-scenes restorative remedy. The dose in either case is four drops on the tongue.

....

Now, back to Jeremy. To put this lovely young man in perspective let me give you a little of his background. Jeremy was 33 years old and had just been promoted to a fairly senior position with a stockbroking firm in the city. He was training for the iron-man competitions and was, as you can imagine, in very good shape. Jeremy was feeling very stressed trying to cope with the immense learning curve of his new position.

I asked Jeremy to describe his diet in detail – giving me a day in the life of his stomach, so to speak. He began the day with a bowl of muesli with milk and a cup of coffee, followed by a cafe latte and fruit for morning tea. Lunch was either a toasted cheese and ham or a chicken and avocado sandwich, and his mid-afternoon snack was a 'sports drink' (used by many as a pick-me-up) plus a muesli bar or some chocolate. From Monday to Thursday dinner was normally quite healthy, consisting of either chicken or fish and steamed vegetables, or else a stir-fry of similar ingredients, with yoghurt or, occasionally, ice-cream for dessert. Unfortunately dinner on the weekends were not so exemplary. Jeremy usually had either takeaway pizza, fish and chips or curry and rice, often washed down with far too much beer on Saturday night.

Jeremy had a long history of antibiotic use. He had been on antibiotics to treat adult acne for most of his 20s, and still resorted to the occasional prescription when he had a bad outbreak. Zinc is the key mineral used to treat skin conditions, and, interestingly, when I tested his zinc status, it was virtually non-existent. (Clinical trials have shown zinc to be more effective in treating extreme acne cases than the powerful drug isotretinoin.) Also, remember the connection between a zinc deficiency and diarrhoea.

Naturopathic diagnostic tools, which always include a tongue, nail and iris analysis, threw more light on this case. Jeremy's tongue was lightly coated with a white film, indicating gut flora imbalance, and his iris showed a distinct predisposition to lymphatic congestion. When I questioned Jeremy further, I discovered that he had suffered from recurrent episodes of tonsillitis as an adolescent. And finally, not surprisingly, Jeremy's nail analysis showed the tale-tale zinc defiency signs of pronounced white flecks.

My first measure to resolve Jeremy's diarrhoea was to ask him to eliminate all dairy products from his diet for six weeks. (The puffiness he had below his eyes is a common symptom in those with a cow's milk sensitivity.) This did not go down too well. Jeremy was addicted to milk, and sometimes drank up to half a litre after training. This fact is enough to make any naturopath suspicious: patients who love milk and cheese nearly always test positive for an allergic response to dairy. When I pass young men in the street slurping from cartons of flavoured milk, it takes all my self control to refrain from marching them off immediately to the nearest lab to test for a dairy allergy. And, I might add, milk is for babies **not** grown men. However, I do not feel this advice would be graciously received!

I also asked Jeremy to: replace all caffeine-containing beverages (coffee and sports drinks) with either meadowsweet tea or water; not to eat any spicy or fatty foods; start the day with a generous teaspoon of slippery elm bark powder mixed into water, taken before breakfast; and have a small bowl of soy yoghurt with slippery elm powder, grated apple and a dollop of Manuka honey each night before bed. To relax the nervous system and soothe the bowel, I prescribed a herbal *medicine mixture of nervine tonics and anti-spasmodic herbs, to be taken twice a day with meals. To replenish his depleted bowel flora, I gave Jeremy a probiotic capsule containing L. acidophilus, B. breve and S. thermophilus, to be taken twice a day before meals. Last, I recommended a strong B-plus-C vitamin complex, designed to treat adrenal exhaustion. (This formula, due to the B vitamin, would also stimulate the production of friendly bowel flora.) To address his acute zinc deficiency, we started immediately on an industrial-strength, liquid zinc supplement, to be taken twice a day in water.*

Although Jeremy initially had a few hiccups with the diet, mainly giving in to milk cravings, once we found a soy milk he found palatable we were on our way. (All soy milks are not created equal! Choose a soy milk made with whole organic soy beans, filtered water, a little canola oil and no malt, sugar or salt.) Within two weeks, Jeremy's stools were much firmer, with only the occasional bout of stress-related diarrhoea, and the 'urgent' episodes had all but gone. After six weeks, Jeremy was feeling much more relaxed, his bowel had completely settled down, and the white coating on his tongue had disappeared. As an added bonus, his skin was blemish free, a result of the probiotic supplement, dietary changes and adequate zinc levels.

9

ADVERSE FOOD REACTIONS:
ALLERGIES, SENSITIVITIES AND INTOLERANCES

Food allergies (also known as sensitivities) and intolerances are major culprits when it comes to a broad range of gastrointestinal disorders. In fact, 'irritable bowel syndrome' (IBS) is, in some medical circles, referred to as a common *allergic* reaction affecting 20 per cent of the population.

When is a reaction against a food classified as an allergy or a sensitivity, and when is it classified as an intolerance? In practical terms this is a purely academic discussion, since no matter what the classification, if a particular food is causing gastro-intestinal grief, it needs to go. However, there is some confusion about these terms so we had better sort out this tricky terminology before we progress any further

A food *allergy* is an adverse immune reaction to the ingestion of a particular food. It is an inflammatory response involving the production of antibodies, either IgE or IgG antibodies. There are two types of food allergies. Type 1 hypersensitivity reaction (also known as an 'immediate' reaction) is an IgE-mediated response and is usually detected with the skin-prick test or a blood test (RAST). The IgE antibody, concentrated in the lung, skin and cells of the mucous membrane, releases chemicals in an *immediate* reaction to a certain food that characteristically produces the flare-and-wheal-like symptoms resulting in itching, redness and rash. This type of food allergy occurs in only 2 per cent of adults and is often seen in combination with eczema or asthma; dairy, wheat, egg, peanut and soy elicit most responses. In extreme cases an IgE allergic response can result in anaphylactic shock. The second type of food allergy, an IgG-antibody response, is far more common. It is often referred to as a 'delayed' hypersensitivity reaction or food sensitivity. It is diagnosed by a blood test, where the blood is challenged with up to 93 different foods and IgG antibodies are noted against each one. This common type of food allergy is believed to occur in people with chronic health conditions, such as IBS, chronic fatigue syndrome (CFS) and fibromyalgia.

Sufferers of undiagnosed food allergies or intolerances feel unwell for most of the time. Except in those rare cases of an immediate IgE allergic response, most people are unable to associate their poor health with an offending food. A study in the *Journal of Clinical Medicine* in 2005 reported that eliminating all foods in which a prior sensitivity was detected by raised IgG antibodies, resulted in a significant improvement in IBS symptoms; that is, abdominal pain, constipation, diarrhoea, flatulence, nausea, gastric reflux. (Australia has the highest rate of allergies – airborne, climatic and food – in the world.)

A food *intolerance*, on the other hand, has nothing to do with the immune system. A particular food elicits a gut-related symptom, without a corresponding formation of an antibody. Lactose intolerance, where the enzyme to break down milk sugar is missing or in short supply, fits into this category of bothersome reactions to food.

Signs and symptoms of food allergies

Allergic reactions are commonly, but not exclusively, felt somewhere along the many metres of our gastrointestinal tract (GIT). Gut-related symptoms can include abdominal pain, bloating, diarrhoea, nausea and constipation. Non-gut-related symptoms include:

- sinusitis
- post-nasal drip
- joint pain
- migraine
- headache
- fatigue
- frequent urination
- asthma
- food cravings
- skin conditions such as eczema, psoriasis and urticaria

- itchy skin and throat
- blue or dark circles beneath the eyes
- fluid retention
- flushed face or ears after eating
- rapid heartbeat and excessive sweating.

In addition (yes, there's more!), symptoms specific to the brain and nervous system include:
- irritability
- dizziness
- mental exhaustion
- poor concentration and memory
- attention deficit disorder (ADD) and attention deficit/hyperactivity disorder (ADHD)
- insomnia.

An exhausting and debilitating collection of reactions that's for sure, but definitely not insurmountable. The key is to clearly identify the offending foods, eliminate them, heal the gut and then challenge by reintroducing the offending food. This is an important point because, as time passes, adverse food reactions can change. Strict adherence to a program of gastrointestinal repair frequently results in a diminished sensitivity to previously allergenic foods. (Children's responses to foods change as they 'outgrow' some of their food allergies or intolerances.) So it is vital to continually assess, challenge and check for new, altered or vanquished food sensitivities. In a moment we will see how we go about this. First, though, let's look at the rather frustrating relationship between food allergies and desire!

Food cravings

Another reason many people find it difficult to associate a particular food with their poor health is that they often crave the very foods they are allergic to. They experience momentary pleasure after consuming the allergenic food because endorphins, such as adrenalin and cortisol, are released that stimulate the 'pleasure and reward' area of the brain. (Adrenalin increases the pulse rate, which is a good way to detect a food allergy. See 'Pulse Test', page 109.) In order to prolong this pleasurable sensation, we continue to eat the foods responsible for this reaction.

Dairy and wheat, not surprisingly, are most frequently associated with this food-addiction response. An enzyme deficiency makes some individuals especially prone to feeling 'spaced out' after eating grains and dairy products. Peptides found in gluten (wheat), called gluteomorphins, and casomorphins from casein (dairy) are uncannily similar to our brain's own endorphins. If these peptides are not broken down by our intestinal enzymes they can exert powerful mental reactions and behaviour. With this sort of biochemical complexity, it is easy to see why adverse reactions to food are so difficult to pinpoint!

Food allergy detection

SKIN-PRICK TEST

As mentioned, the skin-prick test or blood test (RAST) is used to test for immediate, sometimes life-threatening, allergic responses to food – it detects the presence of IgE antibodies. This type of test is commonly used where certain foods are suspected of triggering conditions such as sinusitis, asthma and some skin conditions.

BLOOD TEST FOR SENSITIVITIES

I frequently ask my clients to undertake a blood test to determine possible food sensitivities. This is used to detect an IgG-antibody reaction, which is a very accurate way of determining gut-related food sensitivities. It is a lengthier test that also looks for delayed reactions, and tests against a wider range of foods. (RAST often tests against groups of foods, such as all dairy, whereas the IgG blood test will test against different types of dairy, i.e. cows, goats or sheep). In the years I have been in practice, I have never had one come back with a nil result. Ninety-five per cent of food allergy tests come back positive to dairy, pineapple, cola nut (Coke!), yeast and wheat. This tells us something. The well-documented connection between allergy and addiction explains why many people fill their shopping trolleys with frighteningly large numbers of Coke bottles.

I use this method when there have been many years of poor health. Some clients have already undergone numerous diagnostic and invasive exploratory tests, such as gastroscopies, colonoscopies, ultrasounds and exhaustive blood tests, all of which have returned negative or all-clear results. These clients have more often than not, already undertaken numerous self-inflicted food elimination and challenge trials to no avail. They have had enough, and want, quite understandably, a quick, definitive answer to their chronic gut disorders. Giving these clients yet another list of 'do not eats' or another battery of tests will only cause more stress, and we now know what that can do to our guts. So off they go for a quick prick of the arm, donating a little blood, for which they will receive a scientifically based, definitive list of foods to which they have elicited an immune response. Easy and relatively painless.

Most clients have on average six to ten food allergies, but some unfortunate clients, and I should emphasise these are in the minority, come back with a long list of offending items. One client actually had 62. Out of a potential 95 that's not good. Further testing did however reveal coeliac disease and, not surprisingly, a very leaky gut.

When presented with their results, the majority of clients are relieved to finally discover what *exactly* is disturbing their gut. And I must say, far better to know than not to know. This blood test takes the guesswork out of the rather complex area of food allergies, and it often means that foods which have been avoided for years, 'just in case' they are the villains, can be happily reintroduced. (On this point, if at one stage in your quest for a pain-free GIT you have been told you have a yeast, or dairy or anything else allergy, never accept this as gospel. I see far too many patients who have unnecessarily been avoiding whole groups of food because they were told 20 years ago to delete them.)

Your naturopath can organise the IgG-antibody blood test for you (its correct title is the enzyme linked immuno-sorbent assay test [ELISA]).

PULSE TEST

If you suspect you may have a food allergy, there are a few simple methods that *you* can implement at home to determine if this is the case. Pulse testing is not time consuming, can be performed in the privacy of your own home, and is remarkably accurate and very inexpensive!

In this test it is necessary to abstain from a particular food for at least a few days, and preferably for a month. Before eating that food again, take your pulse at rest, counting beats per minute. Eat the food (by itself) and then after five minutes take your pulse at rest and again ten minutes later. If your pulse is elevated by more than 10 beats per minute, this indicates a strong likelihood of a food allergy or intolerance. (A food allergy can cause the release of the stress hormone adrenalin, which usually causes a rise in the pulse rate.)

FOOD ELIMINATION AND CHALLENGE TEST

Another exercise you can do at home is the 'elimination and challenge' test.

If you suspect food allergies may be causing or contributing to your gut discomfort, but cannot clearly identify the culprit or culprits, the best course of action is an elimination and challenge test. You need to avoid the suspected food for six weeks. This means total avoidance, not one iota of the offending food is permitted, then reintroduce the food after six weeks of exclusion. If allergic, your symptoms should return within the first 24 hours of consuming the suspected food.

Part one: elimination of common allergens

A standard group of suspect foods are eliminated over a six-week period. One food from each excluded group is challenged separately and a diet and symptom diary is kept so that problem foods are clearly identified. Foods to avoid include: dairy, wheat, yeast, eggs, corn, soy, peanuts, oranges, tomato, food additives, coffee, alcohol, oils and fats (except for the essential fatty acids [EFAs]).

Before you throw your hands up in horror and in a trembling tone mutter 'But what is left to eat?' remain calm, plenty of options are left! All fruits except tomatoes and oranges; all vegetables; most proteins, including meat, poultry, fish, beans and legumes (except soy); all nuts, except peanuts; all seeds; and all grains except wheat or corn.

Permitted grains include oats, rice, millet, barley, rye, quinoa and amaranth. However, if you wish to test an allergy to gluten, then gluten-containing grains including wheat, oats, rye and barley need to be struck off the list for a short time as well. Keep in mind that bulgar, couscous, spelt and kamut are wheat-derived or wheat-related and therefore contain gluten. (See appendices 10 and 11 for sample menus for elimination diets, including gluten-free guidelines.)

Part two: challenge diary

The food challenge process occurs once the elimination diet has been adhered to for at least six weeks. Eat only one of the restricted foods on a particular day, in conjunction with your allowable foods. Eat the challenged food at breakfast, lunch and dinner. Keep careful records of the foods eaten and note in a diet diary all symptoms observed (see Appendix 12 for a food challenge diary you can copy). Food challenges occur for one day and any symptoms on that day as well as the next day are noted. Once challenged the food is withdrawn until all other foods are challenged. A full day should elapse before another food is challenged. As well as recording symptoms, you may wish to perform the pulse test, discussed previously, after the challenged food is eaten.

Lactose intolerance

Human beings really are a little illogical at times. Consider this: most mammals once weaned stop drinking milk, but humans continue to drink milk (and not even human milk!) well after infancy and into adult life. Milk consumption often causes gut problems because the lactose-digesting enzyme, lactase, reaches its maximum levels in the human intestinal lining shortly after birth, and then slowly declines, with a relatively low level stabilising between two to five years of age. This is a very logical, very clever biochemical adjustment by our bodies. Why produce an enzyme when it is no longer needed? It's a waste of precious bodily resources. Once most mammals are weaned, they never again encounter lactose in food. Therefore no need having an enzyme to digest it.

The majority of the world's population is lactose-intolerant, with the highest percentages occurring in Asian and black ethnic groups. The great biochemist Harold McGee aptly noted: 'It turns out that adult lactose intolerance is the rule rather than the exception: lactose-tolerant adults are a distinct minority on the planet.'

Lactose intolerance is a result of a shortage not an absolute deficiency of the enzyme lactase, and symptoms are caused by undigested and unabsorbed milk sugar fermenting in the small intestine. Acting osmotically, lactose draws between 150 and 1000 ml of water into the intestine, causing abdominal cramping, nausea, bloating, gas and diarrhoea. Lactose intolerance has also been implicated in depression, as the unabsorbed lactose in the gut decreases the availability of serotonin.

Lactose intolerance is, fortunately, not the same as cow's milk allergy, and small milligram amounts are quite safe. It takes a lot of lactose – tens of grams in fact, not milligrams – to produce symptoms. To give you an idea, milk is 10 per cent lactose, therefore a 200 ml serving of milk contains 20 g of lactose. Most lactase-deficient adults can consume this amount of milk a day without any symptoms. Another bonus for dairy-loving adults is that cheese contains little or no lactose (I can hear a collective sigh of relief), and the friendly bacteria in yoghurt generate lactose-digesting enzymes that get to work in the small intestine.

It is fascinating to note that the little lactase (lactose-digesting enzymes) we do have actually decreases during inflammation. Is it any wonder then that most of us go completely off our dairy products when ill. Our body tells us what to do, if we listen attentively.

Lactose intolerance is frequently observed in coeliac patients. The lactase enzyme lives in the intestinal villus cells (which have microscopic hair-like projections); gluten in the diets of those who suffer from coeliac disease stunt the villus cells – meaning less surface area and therefore decreased numbers of lactose-digesting enzymes. Lactose intolerance is diagnosed by a challenge test using 50 g of lactose.

Fructose malabsorption

Fructose, also called levulose, is a simple sugar found in many fruits as well as honey, wheat and some vegetables.

Fructose has the same chemical formula as glucose but the atoms are arranged in a different structure. Both fructose and glucose are simple monosaccharides while table sugar, by comparison, is a disaccharide – it is made up of a glucose and fructose joined together.

For a small but growing number of the population there is a direct relationship between fructose intolerance and bowel discomfort – particularly, altered bowel frequency. Fructose malabsorption is when the absorption of fructose, which occurs in the small intestine, is impaired. Unabsorbed fructose in the small intestine can cause some rather painful abdominal symptoms. In its unabsorbed state it moves through to the large intestine where bacteria use it as a food source. When bacteria digest fructose it can cause stomach bloating, wind, abdominal pain, loose stools and/or constipation. Over recent years, I have seen an increasing number of cases of fructose-related gut problems.

The only valid method for diagnosing fructose malabsorption is a hydrogen breath test. Clients who limit their daily fructose intake after a positive result to the breath test experience almost immediate relief, with symptoms disappearing overnight. If you suspect that fructose is causing your abdominal symptoms, first try deleting all the high-fructose foods; if symptoms resolve or are minimised, then a fructose malabsorption is highly likely. This diagnosis can be confirmed by the breath test, which normally requires a referral to a gastroenterologist.

Foods most likely to cause problems are: apples, pears, honey, fructose, guava, persimmon, lychee, watermelon, mango, pawpaw, coconut cream, corn syrups and fructo-oligosaccharides (such as psyllium husks; see Chapter 6, Gut flora: Getting the balance right). Fruit juice, dried fruit and tinned fruit in 'natural' juice will also be problematic.

Other seemingly unrelated foods that are also high in dietary fructans are: wheat* (a culprit yet again; whole-meal flour contains more fructose than white flour because wheat germ and bran contain sucrose), leeks, onion (particularly high), green beans, asparagus, spring onion and chicory. Fructose is also widely used as a food additive; best to check all manufactured products.

Note: see Appendix 13 for a comprehensive list of foods that contain wheat.

10

COELIAC DISEASE AND GLUTEN SENSITIVITY

Coeliac disease (sometimes called gluten-sensitive entero-pathy or sprue) is a disorder of the small intestine caused by an immune response to gluten, the protein found in some grains; namely, wheat, rye, barley and oats. In other words, it is a gluten intolerance and it has a clear genetic predisposition. The ingestion of gluten by susceptible individuals causes abnormalities of the small intestine. The antibodies formed against the gliadin proteins (gluten) attack the villi cells in the lining of the intestine, flattening the intestinal mucosa and inhibiting the absorption of nutrients. This produces a variety of symptoms, including malnutrition, diarrhoea and anaemia, and in young children, if not caught early, a failure to thrive. Coelic disease is increasing in prevalence, as is gluten sensitivity, a subclinical form of the disease, both of which frequently go undiagnosed.

Coeliac disease is diagnosed by a blood test and then confirmed by a small-bowel biopsy. The blood test will reveal elevated anti-gliadin or endomysial antibodies, and the biopsy will confirm damage to the intestinal mucosa. (The anti-gliadin antibodies screening test [AGA] requires recent dietary exposure by the person being tested to achieve an accurate result. The endomysial antibody test [EMA] looks for the genetic marker associated with coeliac disease, which is not dependent on gluten in the diet. Both tests can produce false negative or false positive results; therefore, a small-bowel biopsy is recommended if symptoms and screening test indicate coeliac disease.)

The malabsorption of essential nutrients, such as iron, folate, zinc, calcium and fat-soluble vitamins results in iron-deficient anaemia, folate deficiency and reduced bone density. Many coeliacs also have a lactose deficiency and some are found to suffer from osteoporosis as well as anaemia. It is a very serious condition, and can be diagnosed at any stage in life, from early childhood to adulthood.

People diagnosed with coelic disease must strictly avoid all foods that contain gluten. Gluten is found in wheat, rye, barley and oats, and, of course, all wheat-related grains: couscous, spelt, bulgur and kamut. Some forms of wheat are more likely to trigger an autoimmune response than others. Durum wheat, traditionally used to make pasta, has a greater gluten rating than other wheat flours. Hidden sources of wheat/gluten include stamps, envelopes, crayons, play dough and medicines (see Appendix 14, A guide to gluten). Grains that are gluten-free and therefore perfectly safe to consume are rice, corn, millet, buckwheat, quinoa, amaranth, sorghum and teff.

Signs and symptoms of coeliac disease

Commonly experienced signs and symptoms of coeliac disease include abdominal discomfort, bloating, paleness, fluid retention, fatigue and alternating bouts of constipation and diarrhoea. In medical circles the classic coeliac patient is described as 'thin and pot-bellied with steatorrhoea' (steatorrhoea is when there is an excess amount of fat in the stool, causing floating stools). Classic signs in infants are impaired growth, diarrhoea (stools are often foul smelling) and abdominal distention. A general sense of weakness and fatigue are due to the poor absorption of nutrients; especially iron, vitamin B12 and folate. Liver abnormalities are also common. Other signs strongly associated with nutritional deficiencies include mouth ulcers and cracks at the corner of the mouth, erosion of dental enamel, hair loss and an itchy skin rash (called *Dermatitis herpetiformis*, see page 119), which is characterised by the eruption of small blisters.

However, we need to be careful because many people who have coeliac disease do not match this 'typical' picture. They have *no* gut symptoms and some, in fact, have no recognisable signs. They are referred to as 'the silent presenters'. Consequently, coeliac disease is often diagnosed quite late in life, or else misdiagnosed completely due to sharing similar symptoms with a wide range of gut disorders; namely, that unhelpfully named irritable bowel syndrome (IBS), and even chronic fatigue syndrome (CFS).

Dermatitis herpetiformis is often referred to as 'coeliac disease of the skin', while coeliac disease is referred to as 'coeliac disease of the gut'. It is a very itchy skin rash distinguished by the eruption of small papules or blisters. These blisters cause a burning, stinging sensation and often occur in crops, which take up to seven to ten days to lose their itchiness, and then begin to crust. The IgA antibodies, produced by the mucous membranes (of the nose, throat, lungs and gut) in response to gluten, circulate in the blood stream and settle in the skin causing an intense reaction. It is currently believed that oats do not cause *Dermatitis herpetiformis*.

Are oats safe for coeliacs?

This is a very well-debated and complex issue, with some researchers coming down on the side of oats and others positively banning this otherwise benign and nutritious grain. Oats definitely contain gluten; although, it does appear that the gluten in wheat is far more problematic than the gluten in oat. Studies show that moderate consumption of oats does not seem to initiate autoimmune response and subsequent intestinal damage. I recommend an individual assessment for coeliacs; for instance, if after a controlled period of moderately consuming oats a colonoscopy revealed further villi damage, then total avoidance would be necessary.

Treatment for coeliac disease

If you suspect that a gluten intolerance may be accountable for your gut-related symptoms and you have been avoiding these grains for a while, then prior to taking a blood test it is crucial to expose yourself to a little gluten. The elimination of gluten from the diet can have profound effects, and will make a firm diagnosis tricky. No need to go on a happy-go-lucky gluten party, however, only small amounts are necessary. Some people with coeliac disease are extremely sensitive to gluten, so gluten-enrich your diet with care! If you have been living a gluten-free life for months or years, it is advisable to eat it for at least a month before testing in order to allow your body time to make antibodies against it.

An indisputable diagnosis of coeliac disease often comes as quite a shock, and initially it takes a concentrated effort to stick to a gluten-free diet. However, the symptom-free life that quickly follows a coeliac-friendly diet inspires compliance, and is a huge motivation to maintain tight vigilance. The increased mental clarity is one of the first things that clients note. This makes sense as we know that the gluten in grains can latch onto endorphin receptors in the brain, causing a mental fog, poor speech co-ordination and even depression. Fortunately, there is a wide range of gluten-free products on the market, and more and more cafes are offering gluten-free meals. There are even a few cafes catering exclusively to those on gluten-free, dairy-free or wheat-free diets. However, try not to choose gluten-free alternatives of products you would not have previously consumed. This is a mistake that many recently diagnosed patients sometimes fall into. Just because there are some delicious looking gluten-free cakes or biscuits on the shelves of your local health food shop or cafe does not mean you are entitled to them! If you did not eat these types of foods before your diagnosis, now is not the time to start filling your kitchen cupboards and then tummies with sugary, high-fat 'substitute' treats. The best path to take is a healthy well-balanced diet with the occasional treat. Just like the rest of us.

It is extremely important, when following a gluten-free regime, to ensure adequate fibre intake. Too many gluten-free breads and pasta are seriously deficient in this area, so pay strict attention to your fibre count (see Appendix 8, Fibre figures). Focus on whole grains – that means using all parts of the grain – such as brown rice, buckwheat kernels, corn and rolled millet. Liberally sprinkle your meals with linseeds, sunflower and pumpkin seeds to further, deliciously enhance your fibre intake and ensure a smooth, pain-free transit through the bowel zone.

A strict gluten-free diet is crucial for coeliacs to achieve long-term good health, because their condition predisposes them to some very serious diseases – the incidence of which can be hugely reduced by following a gluten-free diet. Diabetes, thyroid disease, liver disease, small bowel carcinoma and cardiomyopathy are more common in coeliacs than the general population.

SUPPLEMENTS

For the first few months following diagnosis it is crucial to take a few basic supplements. For most coeliacs, absorption of key nutrients could have been impaired for quite some time, and until a gluten-free diet is undertaken absorption will continue to be compromised. So, at the very least, a good-quality multi-vitamin containing adequate amounts of all the B vitamins, potassium, magnesium, iron and calcium should be taken daily. You will recall from our study of the gastrointestinal tract (GIT) that saliva is replete with amylase, the carbohydrate-digesting enzyme. Coeliacs, especially, need to chew all food properly – the first step in achieving ideal digestion and absorption. Two additional supplements that I would prescribe at the initial stage after diagnosis are: oral enzymes, which assist in the breakdown and, even more importantly for coeliacs, the absorption of dietary nutrients; and a good-quality probiotic, which improves digestion, repairs intestinal mucosa and stimulates the gut's immune system.

As most gluten-sensitive individuals have compromised absorption of fats, I recommend lacing their diet liberally with Omega 3 and Omega 6 essential fatty acids (EFAs), such as oily fish and flaxseed oil; and vitamin E (a fat-soluble vitamin) also needs to be taken as a supplement (the best form are those that contain the natural d-alpha tocopherol vitamin E). Coeliacs are frequently found to be deficient in vitamin B12, which is primarily absorbed in the ileum, the last portion of the small intestine. Thus a sub-lingual (under the tongue) B12 supplement at a dose of 500–1000 mcg in addition to a multi-vitamin should be taken each day. (A clinical sign of a B12 deficiency is when a tongue is red and beef-like in appearance, and clients often report burning or soreness, particularly on the front portion of the tongue.) Zinc at the very best of times is difficult to absorb, and, not surprisingly, most people with coeliac disease are found to be very deficient in this crucial mineral. I always submit my coeliac patients to the zinc taste test (see page 161), and, to this day, have never had a gluten-intolerant patient pass. So please check your zinc levels if you have coeliac disease.

Many patients with coeliac disease are prone to anaemia and osteoporosis. If anaemic, I would recommend iron supplementation using iron diglycinate or ferrous fumerate, 15 mg three times a day and recheck iron levels within three weeks. Do not take inorganic iron supplements and never use ferrous sulphate, it is irritating to the gut and causes constipation. If osteoporitic, a calcium supplement containing calcium citrate or calcium hydroxyapatite plus the co-factors of magnesium, copper, manganese, boron, zinc, vitamin D3 and vitamin K should be taken. It is best to be taken in split dosages with the majority taken before bed (e.g. one 250 mg tablet at breakfast, one with dinner, two before bed). This will ensure a total intake of 1000 mg elemental calcium a day.

Sub-clinical gluten sensitivity (or non-coeliac gluten intolerance)

Many patients who notice a seemingly irrefutable connection between gluten-containing foods and their abdominal symptoms can, strangely, return a negative blood-test result for coeliac disease. It is possible to have the physiological and neurological symptoms of coeliac disease without abnormalities of the small-intestinal mucosa being detected in a biopsy. Over the years I have had numerous clients' blood tests return positive results for IgG antibodies to gluten-containing grains, yet without a corresponding positive in their blood tests for coeliac disease. It is possible to have a response to the gluten-containing component of grains without full-blown coeliac disease. Why is this so?

Gluten production has increased considerably in the past 20 years or so, making gluten one of the cheapest industrial proteins. Not surprisingly, therefore, we find it sneaking into every manner of food (even meat products) and non-food products (cosmetics), resulting in an increased likelihood of exposure to gluten for the population as a whole, and for coeliacs in particular. Since there is evidence that premature exposure to gluten increases the risk of developing coeliac disease or gluten sensitivity, the insidious nature of gluten is troubling to say the least. Indeed, gluten sensitivity is becoming so common that it is being referred to as a 'clinical chameleon' and even the 'scurvy of the twenty-first century'.

Before moving on, it is worth pondering the effects of an overdose of a single food. If an overdose of a single vitamin such as vitamin C can result in abdominal cramping and/or diarrhoea, then surely it is logical to assume that an overdose of refined ingredients, namely wheat, could be similarly damaging – and the cause of many health problems in our whole society? The increasing incidence of wheat allergies, dairy intolerance, coeliac disease and diabetes is mounting evidence that our dietary choices are seriously unbalanced and totally contrary to our physiological requirements.

Symptoms and treatment of sub-clinical gluten sensitivity

Common symptoms of sub-clinical gluten sensitivity include: mouth ulceration and gastrointestinal disturbances, such as abdominal cramps, flatulence, diarrhoea and nausea. Reactions are often dose-dependant and management consists of reducing gluten to a level required for symptoms to subside, this varies according to individual sensitivity.

Compared to coeliac disease, nutritional deficiency is not so common in gluten sensitivity as there is no damage to the small intestine. However, years of avoiding certain grains and other foods to get to the bottom of this digestive dilemma will have resulted in some level of nutrient deficit, mainly magnesium and the B-group vitamins. This accounts for the symptoms of fatigue and anxiety frequently experienced by those with gluten sensitivity.

11

LEAKY GUT SYNDROME

The mucosal lining of the small intestine acts as a barrier against the penetration of toxic compounds, large undigested food molecules and bacteria. This leak-proof lining, which is only one cell layer thick and can be easily damaged, is thrown into folds, which vastly increases its surface for digestion and absorption.

We can wear away the lining of our gut mucosa by a variety of means: food allergies, alcohol, stress, dietary deficiencies, aspirin, drugs (especially the non-steroidal anti-inflammatory drugs), parasitic infection and chemotherapy. (I always prescribe glutamine to my clients undergoing chemotherapy. It protects the gut lining and also helps to decrease the possibility of nausea and mouth ulceration.)

A constant barrage of regularly consuming foods we are allergic to, washed down with multiple cups of coffee or a few glasses of wine, together with the occasional period of stress and anxiety will certainly guarantee a gut lining that is worn away and overly porous. Chronic stress can induce dysfunction of the intestinal wall in the ileum and colon by decreasing the protective mucus, increasing membrane permeability and altering the cells of this delicate lining. This allows small food particles to diffuse through the intestinal wall and enter the bloodstream – creating an unhealthy situation and resulting in a fatigued and uncomfortable individual.

Increased permeability of the gut lining can stimulate inappropriate immune responses to food and to normal gut flora; bacterial toxins and dietary gluten may cause an inflammatory reaction in the gut and the bloodstream, in some cases triggering a variety of autoimmune diseases. There is some recent scientific speculation that rheumatoid arthritis and leaky gut are linked. Certainly, I have found in the clinical setting that healing the gut of my rheumatoid arthritic patients resulted in decreased inflammation, in proportion with the reduction of gut permeability, and inordinate pain relief.

The greater the permeability, the greater the chance of secondary chronic disease. For example, when the gut mucosa is seriously disturbed, various (toxic) substances have an easy passage to the liver. All substances that originate from bacterial action in the gut and cross the intestinal mucosal lining must be detoxified by the liver. When the gut is leaky, the liver has to work harder and, if the liver's ability to detoxify is impaired, then more toxins are delivered via the bloodstream to other tissues.

An astounding 10 per cent of the liver's weight is made up of lymphocytes (white blood cells involved in the body's immune system) hence, the liver is a crucial participant in regulating the immune system. Antigens that pass through the permeable intestinal mucosa activate these immune cells in the liver, which trigger inflammatory chemicals. These chemicals travel to other organs, including the brain, and can affect the normal biological responses in the immune, endocrine and nervous systems – which in turn can result in chronic disease. To add insult to toxic injury, when the liver is busy trying to detoxify this additional burden of toxins, it also produces stress by-products – free radicals (i.e., hydrogen peroxide, superoxide). These unwanted molecules damage oxygen-sensitive tissues; that is, the brain, heart, blood, lungs and kidneys. This requires immediate and increased anti-oxidant protection and, of course, rapid and complete gut repair.

Symptoms of a leaky gut

Symptoms caused by intestinal permeability may be experienced solely in the abdomen or may involve the whole body. Symptoms include: abdominal discomfort and bloating, fatigue, joint or muscle pain, headache and skin eruptions. Penetration of the gut wall by unwanted substances can lead to pathological changes in distant organs and tissues. Certain clinical conditions are strongly associated with altered intestinal permeability; these include the inflammatory bowel diseases of Crohn's disease and ulcerative colitis, as well as coeliac disease, arthritis, skin conditions such as eczema and psoriasis, autism, migraine, headache and chronic fatigue syndrome (CFS).

Testing for a leaky gut

There is a simple test, organised by your naturopath, you can do if you suspect a leaky gut. This method of measuring gut permeability was established by Claude Andre, a leading French researcher in this field. It involves drinking a sugary substance and then collecting your urine for six hours thereafter, which is then sent to a laboratory for testing. By ingesting two innocuous sugars, lactulose and mannitol, and monitoring their excretion in the urine over a six-hour period, we are able to determine the extent or presence of a permeable gut mucosa. These sugars are not metabolised by humans and measuring their recovery in the urine accurately reflects the degree of permeability or malabsorption. This test will give a definitive result.

Treatment for a leaky gut

Don't be alarmed if your gut-permeability test result is positive – a leaky gut is very easy to heal. I usually use the amino acid glutamine, which has a natural affinity for the gut mucosa, and frequently combine this with aloe vera, slippery elm and licorice root. All of which have gentle soothing properties designed to ensure a renewed, tight-junctioned healthy gut wall. Raw cabbage juice is also an effective and simple way to treat an inflamed gastric mucosa and heal a leaky gut; hence it is useful for people suffering from Crohn's disease, ulcerative colitis or gastric ulcers. Two glasses of cabbage juice daily will usually do the trick, and it is not unpleasant! The exact mechanism involved in the healing effect of cabbage juice is not entirely understood; however, glutamine is one of its major components. At the same time as taking supplements to heal a leaky gut, a diet low in potential or actual allergens is recommended so that further inflammation is not caused. Healing time can take anywhere from six weeks to six months depending on the severity of the damage.

It is important to take a good-quality anti-oxidant, as a depletion of the anti-oxidant glutathione is common in leaky gut syndromes, often contributing to poor liver function. And, as we have noted, a liver under stress also results in a release of a cascade of free radicals into the bloodstream. The most effective way to raise levels of glutathione in the liver is to administer its precursors, cysteine and methionine. These amino acids are the base substances that our body uses to make glutathione, and are common components of a good-quality anti-oxidant.

12

HALITOSIS:
THE LAST BAD BREATH

Halitosis, or bad breath, is normally caused by a mal-function somewhere along the gastrointestinal tract (GIT) – either a faulty digestive system or poor mouth hygiene. Let's be a bit more specific, the usual suspects in causing halitosis are:

- inadequate digestive enzymes or hydrochloric acid (HCI) production
- imbalance of bowel flora, notably *Bifidobacterium lactis*
- constipation
- poor dental hygiene, especially gum disease
- inadequate saliva production.

Other factors that contribute to bad breath include: nose or throat infections, postnasal drip and heavy-metal poisoning (check for a blue line along the gums for lead poisoning). Foods that can contribute to bad breath include: red meat, anchovies, blue and yellow cheeses, salami, pastrami and tuna. These foods leave oils in our mouths that can hang about in an odorous manner for anything up to 24 hours, and are stubbornly resistant to brushing, flossing and gargling.

Morning breath and other matters of the mouth

Unpleasant breath in the morning is caused by the dramatic decrease in saliva production while we sleep. Saliva helps fight bad breath by keeping bacteria in the mouth under control. Morning breath is worse in people who snore or sleep with their mouths open, as this naturally dries up what little saliva remains. The back of the tongue becomes an ideal collecting depot for minute food particles and dead mouth cells, which attract a frenzied bacterial colonisation – not pleasant or conducive for fresh breath!

Meticulous dental hygiene – that is, flossing thoroughly before brushing, especially at bedtime, helps lessen the dry-mouth bacterial overload. Flossing protects the gums from damage and removes all food remnants, and the less food particles remaining in your mouth at bedtime the better. However, I was amazed recently by a patron at my local cinema who flossed her teeth during the film. Besides being bad manners, I was fearful of being the unwanted recipient of a flying food particle. One should really look in the mirror when flossing!

A dry mouth in the morning is exacerbated by alcohol consumption and some prescribed medications; in particular anti-depressants, hypertension drugs, and colds and flu medications. Diabetes also worsens the condition.

In addition to flossing and brushing thoroughly, an excellent habit to acquire is tongue-scraping, an Ayurvedic tradition (an ancient Indian system of medicine) that has been widely embraced by many Westerners. Use a specifically designed tongue scraper available at most health food stores (it looks at bit like a lightweight horseshoe), or purchase a firm toothbrush and use it solely for this ritual. Gently scrape or brush your tongue from the back to the tip, removing any coating. Rinse your mouth afterwards with water or, even better, water with a few drops of citrus-seed extract, or, alternatively, finish with a gargle of liquid zinc. Both zinc and citrus extract are strong anti-fungals, helping to remove pathogenic organisms with one or two gargles or mouthfuls (studies show that citrus-seed extract has anti-microbial properties). Remember to replace your toothbrush every month, or immediately after an infectious illness, to prevent bacterial buildup. A recent tongue scraping trial reported a 75 per cent reduction in bad breath after using a tongue scraper, and a 45 per cent reduction after tooth brushing.

While on the subject of oral health, loose gums or indeed gum disease benefit from the local application of coenzyme Q10. Simply pierce a capsule and use the liquid as a paste on the affected gums, leave overnight. Additionally, take a 100 mg capsule of coenzyme Q10 each day to increase tissue oxygenation (anaerobic bacteria do *not* thrive in well-oxygenated environments).

A few easy changes to our diet and lifestyle will have our breath fresh and our oral hygiene restored at best within a couple of weeks and at worst a few months. These changes include: increasing consumption of enzyme enhancing foods and decreasing consumption of red meat and dairy, resolving constipation and bowel flora imbalance and adjusting our teeth- and tongue-cleaning techniques.

....

Maxine was 33 years old when she came to see me for treatment for what she thought were three unrelated health concerns: bad breath, constipation and dark circles under her eyes. She had experienced bad breath for quite some time, and was quite tearful when discussing it during our consultation. Maxine worked with young children, who are often brutally honest when it comes to matters of personal hygiene. Clearly, it was a very sensitive issue, and understandably so. She also felt she sweated excessively. The palms of her hands were frequently so clammy that she shunned situations where she may be required to shake hands.

Maxine was sleeping poorly and waking tired most mornings. Her bowel had always been on the sluggish side, but over the past two years it had become progressively worse, and she now rarely had a daily bowel motion.

In Maxine's case her halitosis was caused by chronic

constipation that fluctuated in severity, inefficient digestive enzymes and incompatible food combinations. The dark circles under her eyes supported this diagnosis as they usually indicate a sluggish liver function, which in turn almost certainly guarantees a sluggish bowel. The first step was to get Maxine to have a daily, complete bowel motion.

Maxine's diet looked something like this: no breakfast or just a glass of milk; lunch was a Chinese-style stir-fry of either beef or pork, or else sushi rolls; dinner was red meat, chicken or, occasionally, fish with a maximum of three vegetables. Snacks included dry biscuits, lollies or chocolate and, before bed, Maxine would have another glass of milk. On weekends she often had a 'special souvlaki' consisting of red meat, yellow cheese and yoghurt (ahhhrr – a triple-protein combination!). And, to make matters worse, this combination was normally consumed late at night after an evening of clubbing.

Clearly Maxine's diet contained too much milk, insufficient fresh fruit and vegetables, some poor food combinations and not enough fibre. Milk and red meat were totally banished for the next two weeks. I suggested that Maxine have either a small bowl of very high-fibre muesli or 3–4 tablespoons seed mix moistened with pear or apple juice for breakfast; substitute vegetarian stir-fries for meat-based ones and eat a bitter leafy salad with dinner each night. Sushi was banned. Raw fish and white rice **do not** guarantee regular bowel function or pleasant breath. I asked Maxine to drink dandelion root coffee and to start the day with a gentle liver *stimulant – the old warm-water-and-lemon-juice routine.*

Maxine was not happy about my ban on milk, and felt she would be unable to go without red meat. To encourage her compliance I asked her to keep a diet diary for the entire fortnight between consultations, recording everything she ate as well as noting her bowel function and breath quality. I was hoping that a positive result from the dietary changes would persuade Maxine to stick to the straight and narrow or, more accurately expressed, the bowel-friendly road.

*Maxine was quite an anxious young woman, and I wondered how much her stress levels had contributed to her poor digestive-enzyme production. In Chapter 3, we discussed how the nervous system affects the gut and vice versa. You may recall that serotonin, an important neurotransmitter found in the gut **and** the brain, regulates both our mood and digestive function. Maxine's state of anxiety would have depleted her of serotonin, increasing her stress levels and contributing to her digestive discomfort and unsatisfactory bowel function.*

I prescribed a course of digestive enzyme tablets containing HCl and pancreatic enzymes and some very bitter herbs that would provide some immediate relief with enzyme supplementation as well as kick-start Maxine's own production of digestive enzymes. The rationale behind this is that, when the supplements were removed, Maxine would be happily generating copious amounts of her own HCl without any need of assistance. The dandelion coffee and bitter greens would help this along. In addition, I made up a herbal prescription featuring some of our most effective liver-stimulating herbs, such as St Mary's thistle, globe artichoke and fringe tree, 5 ml to be taken three times a day.

I asked Maxine to gargle and rinse her mouth out with liquid chlorophyll, as well as taking 10 ml twice a day. Chlorophyll is nature's internal deodoriser and is also serendipitously an excellent source of thousands of enzymes. You can make your own liquid chlorophyll by juicing any edible green plant, such as spinach, parsley or sprouts, or combine powdered green barley with kelp. As mentioned, I felt there was a strong connection between Maxine's inadequate production of pancreatic enzymes and her stretched nervous system; so, to kill two birds with one stone I prescribed a nutritional supplement to boost serotonin levels, featuring the amino acid tryptophan and various co-factors, namely vitamins B1, 2, 3 and 6, folic acid, magnesium and zinc, to be taken on an empty stomach three times a day.

I am pleased to report that within two weeks, Maxine's bowel function had improved markedly, at this stage mainly due to her dietary changes, and there was a noticeable improvement in her breath. Her initial negative response to eliminating red meat from her diet was replaced four weeks later with 'I don't care if I never eat it again'. Such a drastic measure was not required since, within three months of treatment, Maxine's digestion had improved sufficiently that she could eat red meat and hard cheeses without any accompanying distress.

When I sent Maxine on her way, with just the barest of supplements and a request to watch her milk intake in the future, she remarked she no longer liked the taste of milk, finding it to be 'too much like a cow'! This is not uncommon, many clients make the same comment after a period of excluding dairy from their diet.

....

13

THE IMPORTANCE OF DIGESTIVE ENZYMES AND HYDROCHLORIC ACID

'The fate of the nation has often depended upon the good or bad digestion of a Prime Minister.'
— *VOLTAIRE*

Like Voltaire, I frequently wonder how decisions of national importance can be reached by cabinet ministers after they have consumed a large three-course state luncheon of incompatible food combinations eaten in a less than relaxed environment.

Digestive enzymes and gastric juices are essential for the breakdown of foods into smaller nutritional components that can be absorbed and then used by our bodies. An inadequate production of digestive acids and enzymes can lead to a wide range of digestive complaints. Hypochlorhydria is when the amount of hydrochloric acid (HCl) produced by the cells lining the stomach is too low; whereas, pancreatic insufficiency occurs when there are insufficient levels of enzymes (protease, amylase and lipase) manufactured in the pancreas. (You will recall in Chapter 2, when we embarked on our excursion through the gastrointestinal tract [GIT], we discussed the local manufacturers of these important enzymes; namely the stomach and the pancreas.) Unpleasant digestive disorders and even malnutrition can be the result of inadequate digestive enzyme production. Enzyme-deficient diets have also been implicated in heart disease and immune dysfunction.

We have another type of enzyme: metabolic. Metabolic enzymes are responsible for structuring and repairing every cell in our body. The great pioneer of enzyme research Dr Edward Howell suggested that diets low in naturally occurring enzymes force the body to use up its *metabolic* enzymes to digest foods. Shifting enzymes from their metabolic role, such as maintenance of the immune system, waste removal, tissue healing and repair, leaves the body vulnerable and open to many diseases.

Signs and symptoms of hypochlorhydria and pancreatic insufficiency

There are subtle differences in the signs and symptoms of HCI and pancreatic enzyme insufficiency, although deficiencies in either can cause bad breath. Symptoms of a lack of HCI could include:

- upper-abdominal bloating and gas (and belching)
- reflux
- constipation

- feeling full shortly after eating
- poor appetite (the 'I am never really hungry' syndrome)
- broken capillaries on the cheeks (acne rosacea is a type of adult acne characterised by broken capillaries and red pimples, almost exclusively seen in women in the 30–50 age bracket and treated with HCl supplementation)
- vertical splitting of the nails
- food and chemical sensitivity.

Symptoms of pancreatic insufficiency, on the other hand, could include:

- lower-abdominal bloating and gas
- indigestion, normally experienced within about three hours of eating
- constipation alternating with diarrhoea
- foul-smelling stools, possibly containing undigested food particles
- floating stools (due to a large amount of fat in the stool, or too much gas).

Escalating food sensitivities and heartburn are also commonly experienced because of a lack of enzymes or HCl to break down a range of foods. Indeed, it is believed that the peptides generated during the digestion of grains and dairy products, called exorphins, are highly resistant to some enzymes, and may escape digestion altogether in individuals prone to digestive enzyme deficiency. An accumulation of these exorphins in the central and enteric nervous systems is thought to be responsible for the 'spaced out' feeling often experienced by those with food allergies and intolerances.

Optimum enzyme activity is needed to effectively break down the proteins and carbohydrates in a high-fibre diet, otherwise constipation can result. Another consequence of a lack of enzymes is that any undigested carbohydrates are fermented in the colon, creating gas and organic acids; the excess gas causes flatulence and makes stools float. When there are inadequate digestive enzymes, there is nearly always dysbiosis – that is, an imbalance of intestinal flora – which is caused by poor short-chain fatty acid (SCFA) metabolism. You may recall that SCFAs are the principle by-products of the breakdown of carbohydrates. These by-products provide fuel for the manufacture of intestinal flora; they also affect faecal bulk.

Hypochlorhydria can cause an overgrowth of endogenous bacteria in the stomach, small intestine and cecum. A classic symptom of bacterial overgrowth is carbohydrate intolerance, with associated excess gas and bloating. Bacterial overgrowth is particularly problematic for those taking medication to decrease production of gastric HCI or frequently on antibiotic therapy, and especially for the elderly who experience a decrease in HCI production as well as a general decline in digestive enzyme secretion. Keith Eaton, a British allergist who has worked extensively with gut-fermentation syndrome, found that taking amino acid L-histidine (500 mg twice a day) improved gastric-acid production in patients with hypochlorhydria.

Causes of hypochlorhydria and pancreatic insufficiency

Low enzyme and HCl production is usually due to three factors: diet, stress and ageing. Eating habits are major culprits, namely: inadequate chewing, a lack of raw foods, eating too late in the day or eating on the run (remember Maxine), and drinking liquids with meals, which dilutes digestive enzymes. Stress, both emotional and physical, can stunt enzyme production, as the body shuts down 'non essential' functions when under stress. Gastric secretion, for example, is inhibited by rage, fear, pain and unpleasant odours and tastes. As we age we also experience a decline in enzyme secretion – our body parts simply wear out. However, all of these enzyme-reducing factors can be remedied with a few easy lifestyle changes, enzyme supplementation and dietary enhancements.

Treatment of hypochlorhydria and pancreatic insufficiency

How to encourage digestive enzyme production through diet:

- Eat more raw foods. Raw foods contain enzymes that are activated and released during the chewing process. The cooking and processing of food destroys nearly all naturally occurring enzymes. These enzymes initiate the breakdown of food, giving our body a digestive head start.

  According to the 'law of adaptive secretion of digestive enzymes' (see page 151), if some of the food we eat is digested by the enzymes contained in the food, then the body will need to secrete less of its own enzymes. This allows our body to re-direct its energy output from digestion to other important body functions, such as repair and rejuvenation.

  Enhance your diet with a variety of raw, inter-esting salads – and I don't mean lettuce, tomato and cucumber! (*Never* eat cucumber skin, it is very difficult to digest, and be careful eating raw cap-sicum, many people find it extremely difficult to digest, experiencing horrible capsicum-burps for hours afterwards.) While I am on this subject I shall have a quick naturopathic grumble. I get very cross when presented with a salad in a cafe that contains rocket with stalks, limp lettuce, unpeeled cucumber and ice-cold tomatoes. This is sloppy presentation *and* damaging to our digestive systems. Make your own nutritious salad mixes of baby organic rocket, sprouts, beetroot leaves, radicchio, and consider

adding snow peas, celeriac and dandelion leaves.
Add aromatic seeds to further aid digestion; particularly caraway, dill and anise.

- Choose pineapple and papaya for dessert. These
fruits contain bromelain and papain, respectively,
both good sources of digestive enzymes. Make
sure you leave at least one hour before eating,
as fruit should always be eaten on an empty
stomach. (Bear in mind, however, that a high
percentage of the population have a sensitivity to
pineapple. Ninety-nine per cent of food-allergy
tests I conduct in the clinic come back to me
showing an IgG allergy response to this delicious
but problematic fruit.)

- Consume foods rich in enzymes such as fermented
dairy products and soy products; that is, yoghurt,
miso or tempeh. Include at least one serving of
these stomach-friendly foods in your diet daily.
If you have a sensitivity to dairy, choose either
goat, sheep or soy yoghurt. Add miso paste to
soups and casseroles or mix with tofu as a spread,
and drink miso soup prior to meals or as a mid-
afternoon snack.

- Sip apple cider vinegar with meals. One generous
teaspoon of a good-quality, oak-aged apple
cider vinegar in a glass of soda water before
meals, sprinkled with a few caraway seeds is a

delicious aperitif. (It's true! Not quite as pretty as a Campari, but much more therapeutic.) If you cannot tolerate apple cider vinegar, then lemon juice in water will have the same effect. Older readers, in particular, will greatly benefit from the apple-cider-vinegar routine to kick-start production. Make it part of your daily routine.

A simple test you can do at home to determine if you have a HCI deficiency is to take a tablespoon of apple cider vinegar with your main meal. If this improves your symptoms, especially any indigestion, then you can safely assume you have too little stomach acid.

- Eat more bitter foods. Bitter foods that stimulate digestion include bitter green salads, especially chicory, watercress, rocket and radicchio; and dandelion root coffee (always use the roasted dandelion root, rather than the lactose-infused granules).

All of these digestive-enhancing measures should, needless to say, be consumed slowly in a relaxed, unhurried manner and calm environment. Cut your food into small pieces and chew thoroughly (it helps to liberate plant enzymes). It sounds tedious but actually counting the number of times you chew each mouthful creates awareness – establishing better eating habits encourages digestive comfort. (I know,

I can hear you all saying, does this naturopath have a life? In my defence, I shall counter that with: balance creates happiness!) Eating several small meals throughout the day rather than one or two large ones is recommended, as well as taking a few deep abdominal breaths prior to beginning each meal.

Enzyme-enhancing salad

Choose organic vegetables whenever possible (organic vegetables will be richer in all nutrients as well as have increased enzyme power).

> ½ beetroot, scrubbed and grated
> the smaller beetroot leaves, washed
> 1 carrot, scrubbed and grated
> a generous handful alfalfa spouts
> 1 cup bean sprouts
> 2 cups baby rocket leaves
> 1 small radicchio
> 1 small celeriac root, scrubbed and finely julienned
> ½ cup sunflower seeds, lightly dry roasted
> ½ teaspoon caraway seeds
> ½ teaspoon dill seeds or 2 teaspoons fresh chopped dill
> Celtic salt to taste

Dressing
> 2 tablespoons organic extra virgin olive oil

1 tablespoon organic balsamic vinegar
2 tablespoons finely chopped fresh coriander
juice of ½ lemon or lime

Place all the vegetables in a large attractive bowl. (Yes, visual appeal of both ingredients and crockery is important. Think of the difference in experience of consuming pumpkin soup from a polystyrene cup compared to out of your favourite fine china bowl. As humans we respond to beauty.) Combine dressing ingredients in a glass jar and shake well, pour generously over salad. Sprinkle with roasted sunflower and caraway seeds, dill and salt.

ENZYME SUPPLEMENTS – A CAUTIONARY NOTE

A great many digestive enzyme supplements contain pancreatic enzymes from animal sources, mainly pigs. A practice considered by many to be morally questionable, they are often physiologically ineffective and there is some doubt as to whether even an enteric-coated capsule (one that has a protective covering that allows it to reach the intestines intact) can protect animal-based pancreatic enzymes from the highly acidic environment of the stomach. Recent studies suggest that plant enzymes, in comparison to animal enzymes, remain more stable and are more effective across a wide pH range. Plant enzyme supplements are produced cruelty-free and, of course, are suitable for use by vegetarians. To check an enzyme supplement for animal products look for the following key words: porcine, pancreatin, whole pancreas extract or, simply, animal-derived.

HOW TO GET THE MOST FROM YOUR ENZYMES

It is always very important to consider the quality and potential effectiveness of any nutritional supplement, particularly enzymes. They travel a long way and need to arrive intact. Choose products that contain a broad spectrum of enzymes – amylase, protease, lipase and lactase – so that proteins, carbohydrates, dietary fats and lactose are effectively broken down and digested. Other beneficial ingredients would be bromelain and papain (derived from pineapple and papaya, respectively), which are excellent forms of proteolytic enzymes, capable of digesting proteins. Although, be careful if you have a sensitivity to either of these fruits.

Depending on the strength of the capsule and the size of your meal, a general rule of thumb for dosage is two capsules no longer than 30 minutes prior to each meal. They are most effective if taken just before a meal as they will mix with the food and help initiate the digestive process.

At one time naturopaths were worried that supplementation may stunt the body's production of enzymes – the opposite of what we want to achieve. We want to encourage the pancreas to make its own enzymes, not to become lazy and rely on long-term supplementation. However, no need to worry. It appears that some of the enzymes secreted are transported back to the pancreas to be reserved and re-used. Recent studies show that enzyme supplementation conserves the body's own digestive enzymes by contributing to the pool of enzymes available for re-secretion. Very economical. This is known as the 'law of adaptive secretion of enzymes'.

Note: oral supplementation of digestive enzymes is generally without adverse effects in most individuals. However, they are definitely not to be used by anyone with gastric or duodenal ulcers, or with a known hypersensitivity to pineapple or papaya (if bromelain or papain are a component of an enzyme supplement). If any burning sensation occurs after use, discontinue immediately.

MINERALS AND HCI

Mineral therapy is especially suitable for mild hypochlorhydria. Potassium chloride is particulary helpful for encouraging the production of HCI. This mineral is readily absorbed in the stomach and the small intestine, and, as well as producing and maintaining HCI in the stomach, it also helps to regulate pH balance (potassium chloride together with HCI are contained in gastric acid). This twin mineral supplement is effective in cases of indigestion and flatulence, especially after eating fatty meals. It also encourages a healthy appetite after chronic illness or in cases of anorexia. I normally prescribe potassium chloride with sodium phosphate, a supplement known in naturopathic circles as

SPPC. Sodium phosphate is a superb mineral to treat any condition where there is an excessive accumulation of metabolic acid waste (e.g. uric acid, lactic acid) in the tissues, resulting in gout or post-exercise muscle soreness. It is a specific remedy for the gastro-intestinal signs and symptoms of sour-tasting gastric reflux, fat intolerance and odorous stools. Sodium phosphate encourages healthy gallbladder function and prevents the crystallisation of cholesterol in the gallbladder. Not a bad combination, and a very efficient healing tool for digestive distress and sluggishness.

A CASE AGAINST ANTACIDS

There is *no* case for using antacids in any circumstances. Antacids are normally taken to relieve indigestion or heartburn, but, in fact, they make the condition far worse. Long-term use of antacids may result in a variety of chronic digestive disorders: antacids that contain aluminum* compounds can cause constipation, those containing magnesium compounds may cause diarrhoea and sodium bicarbonate-based antacids often result in gas and abdominal distension.

Antacids do *not* assist with gas or bloating. Let's look at how they impact on our digestive process. Four organs are involved in digestion: the stomach secretes HCl to break down protein, and gastric lipase begins the hydrolysis of fats; the pancreas secretes protease, lipase and amylase; and the gallbladder and liver are responsible for the production, storage and secretion of bile. Switching off any one of these essential and interconnected components affects the digestive process. Antacids 'work' by neutralising the acid in the stomach, thereby preventing effective digestion and reducing the absorption of nutrients from our food. In fact, it guarantees the inefficient breakdown of food particles and therefore *exacerbates* abdominal discomfort, not to mention negatively impacting on our nutritional status. Even the healthiest of diets is of little value if we are unable to break down and absorb its nutrients. *Never* use antacids. There are safe and effective herbal remedies, such as: ginger, meadowsweet and peppermint teas; slippery elm powder mixed with water and drunk prior to a meal; or chewing on a few whole anise seeds.

Note: the accumulation of aluminium in the brain is considered a contributing factor in Alzheimer's and Parkinson's diseases, learning difficulties and hyperactivity in children. It can also lead to osteomalacia – a bone-loss disorder.

14

HOW TO OVERCOME
A SLUGGISH METABOLISM

When we speak about our *metabolic rate* we are referring to the rate at which our body burns fuel. As you will
see from this chapter, the thyroid gland plays a major role
in regulating our metabolic rate. The key factor in the
metabolism of fat and other food products is thermogenesis, or the production of body heat through the burning
of energy. When our metabolic rate is slow, less food is
converted into energy and more fat is stored.

A sluggish metabolism *can* lead to weight gain, however, only a very small percentage of overweight people have
a serious metabolic disorder. Weight gain is often due to
excessive calorie input and insufficient energy output. Or
to put it simply, eating too much and not exercising enough.
It is a very easy equation. Humans have strong hunger signals
and weaker satiety signals (genetically designed to accom-
modate periods when food supply was not guaranteed). And
when you combine this biological factor with the pleasure
we derive from eating, the increased food portions served in

cafes and restaurants, and the large 'value sized' packaged meals promoted by supermarkets it is easy to understand why we so frequently override the body's satiety signals! In addition, fats, sugars and food allergies, especially wheat and milk allergies, affect the levels of serotonin in the brain, which can lead to addictive overeating.

Despite all this food, a common cause of a sluggish metabolism and subsequent weight gain is a *nutritional deficiency*! A diet lacking in iodine, tyrosine and zinc, in particular, can ultimately reduce our metabolic rate, which means an increase in fat storage (lipogenesis) and a decrease in the conversion of energy to heat (thermogenesis).

Fat is metabolised within our fat and muscle cells; thus, low-muscle mass is one factor that can reduce our capacity to burn body fat. Additional factors that play a significant role in the rate at which we burn fat and can, therefore, cause cellular dysfunction include: insulin resistance, thyroid hormones, stress levels and toxic loads. In fact, any malfunction at the cellular level may impair fat metabolism. (Other factors that are beyond the scope of this book include sex hormones, inflammation and infections.)

The thyroid gland and thermogenesis

The thyroid gland is located just below the larynx (voice box) and is mainly filled with sacs containing follicles. These follicles manufacture the thyroid hormones: thyroxine, also called T4, and triiodothyronine, or T3. Blood tests for thyroid function normally measure thyroid-stimulating hormones (TSH), which control nearly all aspects of thyroid activity. (If your TSH results are abnormal, T3 and T4 are then measured.) The thyroid hormones regulate basal metabolic rate (BMR = rate-of-oxygen consumption at rest, after fasting overnight), cellular metabolism, growth and development. They increase metabolic rate by stimulating the production of cellular energy. The thyroid hormones regulate our metabolism by stimulating protein synthesis, triglyceride breakdown, increasing cholesterol excretion in bile and the use of glucose for energy production. Therefore an underactive thyroid (hypothyroidism) results in a sluggish metabolism. It is a crucial part of our anatomy, to be treasured and looked after at all times.

Signs and symptoms of hypothyroidism

Signs and symptoms of hypothyroidism include:
- fatigue
- brittle or dry hair, skin and nails
- hair loss
- constipation
- cold intolerance
- decreased concentration
- drooping or swollen eyelids
- difficulty losing weight.

MEASURING YOUR BASAL BODY TEMPERATURE

Our body temperature reflects our metabolic rate. Here is a simple and effective test you can perform in the comfy confines of your own bed to determine if your metabolic rate is sluggish. This test involves measuring your body temperature at rest. The steps to follow are:

1) Place a thermometer close to your bed before going to sleep at night. If using a non-digital thermometer, shake it to below 35 °C.

2) On waking, place the thermometer under your armpit for 10 minutes. Lie still and relax with eyes closed.

3) Record your temperature after 10 minutes.

4) Take your temperature for at least three consecutive mornings, preferably at the same time each day. (Note: Menstruating women should perform this test only on the second, third and fourth day of menstruation.)

5) Take an average of the temperatures.

A body temperature of between 36.4 and 37.1 °C reflects normal thyroid activity, whereas a reading of 36.4 °C or lower may indicate an underactive thyroid. If your temperature indicates the possibility of hypothyroidism, the next step is to have a blood test to measure TSH. However, even if this returns a normal result, you may still have what is referred to as sub-clinical hypothyroidism. And clinical experience supports the fact that there are a lot of people walking around with a less than satisfactory thyroid gland.

Treatment for a sluggish metabolism

Fortunately there are a few simple measures you can take to feed the thyroid and kick-start it into efficient working order again – and boost your metabolic rate.

SUPPLEMENTS

Iodine

A deficiency in iodine needs to be given supplementation priority. The thyroid gland requires iodine (as well as tyrosine, selenium and zinc) to make the thyroid hormones T3 and T4, and although we need only trace amounts of this mineral it is still often found to be lacking in the diets of many people. A contributing factor is that the soils in a considerable number of countries are iodine and zinc deficient. A visible sign of extreme iodine deficiency is a goitre on the neck.

Iodine is especially concentrated in seafood, saltwater fish and kelp. Clients who I suspect are sluggish in the thyroid department are immediately advised (no negotiation entered into!) to sprinkle their vegetables with a generous teaspoon of kelp granules. This is a fantastic way to supplement with iodine without the bother of taking yet another tablet. (Do *not* use kelp powder – very green, very powdery, very sticky on the palate and teeth.) If a therapeutic sprinkling of kelp granules does not hit the spot and you prefer the tablet option (which would be a 1000–1200 mg daily dosage), be sure to take it with plenty of water. I had the most frightful experience with a kelp tablet some time ago, and still find the thought of swallowing one rather off-putting. Kelp tablets are a little coarse or furry in texture and can, if you are not concentrating on the task at hand, get caught in the throat on the way down. Perhaps try the granules first.

Tyrosine

The other nutrients required for a thyroid gland in tip-top condition are, as mentioned, the amino acid tyrosine and the minerals selenium and zinc. Tyrosine attaches to iodine atoms to form thyroid hormones, and low-plasma levels of tyrosine are associated with hypothyroidism. Other symptoms of tyrosine deficiency include: low-blood pressure, low-body temperature, depression, anxiety and restless leg syndrome. Tyrosine is also a precursor to the mood-elevating neurotransmitters norepinephrine and dopamine. A deficiency of norepinephrine in the brain may also, interestingly, result in poor-appetite control and, subsequently, increased body fat. So this amino acid plays a crucial role in maintaining a normal metabolic rate and needs to be addressed in any weight-management program. Good sources of tyrosine include almonds, bananas, dairy products, lima beans, sesame seeds and pumpkin seeds. Daily supplementation with tyrosine is normally 1000 mg, taken as a divided dose on an empty stomach. Be sure to take with the co-factors vitamins B2 and B5, vitamin C and zinc.

Selenium

Selenium is a potent anti-oxidant, capable of inhibiting the oxidation of lipids (fats), preventing the formation of free radicals and certain cancers, protecting the liver from alcoholic cirrhosis and, when combined with zinc and vitamin E, treating prostatic hyperplasia (enlarged prostate). Selenium also plays a key role in the production and conversion of our thyroid hormone T4 to T3. (We now know that both iodine and tyrosine are essential components of T3 and T4.) The enzyme responsible for catalysing the conversion of T4 to T3 (5'-iodothyronin deiodinase) is selenium dependent. In a randomised, placebo-controlled trial, patients were given either 200 mcg of selenium or a placebo for three months. Results indicated that selenium supplementation decreased thyroid gland inflammation as well as improved thyroid hormone levels.

Selenium deficiency has been linked to high-cholesterol levels, frequent infections, pancreatic insufficiency and reproductive sterility. This remarkable mineral is concentrated in meats and grains; the level of selenium is dependent, of course, on the selenium content of the soil where the food is grown or raised. I always feel uncomfortable talking about a cow as a food, and, indeed, why bother a cow when we can obtain rich supplies of selenium from Brazil nuts, brewer's yeast, garlic, seafood, especially salmon and tuna, brown rice and wheat germ. The normal supplemental dose of selenium is 200 mcg. It's best to use selenomethionine, an organic form of supplemental selenium that is more readily absorbable than other forms (such as selenium selenite).

Zinc

Zinc plays the role of the middle man when it comes to the production of thyroid hormones. What follows is a little complex, but it is important to understand the interconnectedness of these minerals. The thyroid-releasing hormone (TRH) found in the hypothalamus of the brain, controls the secretion of TSH, which in turn stimulates the secretion of our thyroid hormones, T3 and T4. In other words, we need zinc to ensure we make and distribute our thyroid hormones.

Zinc is also required for the uptake of the mineral chromium, which as we shall see regulates the absorption of insulin and stabilises blood-sugar levels. Zinc affects prostate gland function, promotes an effective immune system, helps treat and prevent acne, heals wounds and enhances our sense of smell and taste.

Very few of my clients make it through to the end of a consultation without submitting, willingly I might add, to the zinc taste-perception test (zinc tally). Sadly, not many receive an elephant stamp. The test involves holding 10 ml of liquid zinc in the mouth for about 20 seconds, then swallowing the solution and describing the taste. A person's perception can range from 1–4 starting with no specific taste to sweet, sour, salty or metallic. Most clients respond with 'Oh, it tastes just like water', to which I gently reply: 'Unfortunately, that indicates a rather severe zinc deficiency'. I attempt to soften the blow by adding that the soils in Australia are quite low in zinc and it is a difficult mineral to absorb, but not to worry as we can turn this zinc-deficient state around quite quickly with a little liquid zinc supplementation.

Best sources of dietary zinc include pumpkin seeds, sunflower seeds, brewer's yeast, egg yolks, fish, and red meat. However, zinc from many foods is difficult to absorb because compounds called phytates, which are found in grains and legumes and are often good sources of zinc, bind with zinc, blocking its absorption. Combine this with poor levels of zinc in our soil and we have a real possibility of a nationwide zinc deficiency. (If I was prime minister, I would add zinc to the drinking water, ensure every child received an education in sound nutrition and subsidise the production of organic and biodynamic foods. That would solve the zinc problem!)

Zinc absorption is also compromised when taken at the same time as iron supplements, and dairy foods, specifically casein, further inhibit zinc uptake.

Zinc supplementation is best in the form of zinc

sulphate, which comes in a highly soluble liquid form. The dose is dependant on the result of the zinc taste-perception test, but a sensible starting point would be 4 ml taken at a 1:100 dilution twice a day. Retest within two months. It is important that the zinc sulphate supplement contains the co-factors of magnesium and vitamin B6. Avoid supplements containing zinc carbonate or zinc oxide. Although relatively inexpensive when compared to zinc sulphate, it is a false economy as they are poorly absorbed.

Chromium

Insulin is our 'clearance' hormone; that is, it is responsible for clearing glucose from the blood into the body's cells and fat stores. Studies show that many overweight people have higher than normal levels of circulating insulin indicating insulin resistance (also known as syndrome X or metabolic syndrome). This results in abnormal glucose metabolism. The raised levels of glucose slow the breakdown of fat because plenty of available glucose means that the body does not need to utilise stored fat as energy. Subsequently weight-loss is impaired. To make weight loss even more troublesome, raised glucose levels can also cause intense sugar cravings. A double-edged sword. Fortunately, chromium taken as the supplement glucose tolerance factors (GTF) lowers these glucose peaks and the amount of circulating insulin. Thus fat is metabolised faster and weight loss proceeds according to plan.

Glucose intolerance is one of the signs of a chromium deficiency. (Approximately 25–50 per cent of the world's population is deficient in chromium.) If you tend to feel a little shaky and sweaty mid-afternoon or following a refined carbohydrate meal, then you may benefit from chromium supplementation. These are fairly typical symptoms of very low blood-glucose levels or glucose intolerance. A high-sugar diet increases the excretion of chromium in urine by between 10 and 300 per cent.

GTF is made up of mineral chromium, plus its co-factors vitamin B3 and the three amino acids glycine, cysteine and glutamic acid. Take one tablet three times a day (make sure your supplement contains 200 mcg of chromium amino acid chelate or chromium nicotinate). Even better, choose a GTF supplement with the herb gymnema (*Gymnema sylvestre*). This herb is traditionally used in Ayurvedic medicine and its Hindi name is madhunashini, which means 'sugar destroyer'. It blocks the sweet taste of foods, and, more importantly, animal clinical studies show that it increases insulin sensitivity and reduces blood glucose. (Gymnema can also be prescribed by your naturopath as a liquid herbal extract for sweet-cravings and as a sweet taste suppressant. Two ml a day is all that is necessary!)

DIET

A delicious way to include all the abovementioned thyroid-friendly nutrients in your daily diet is to eat:

- Brazil nuts (three Brazil nuts a day provides the daily recommended allowance of selenium)
- fish (not tuna, a 198 g can of tuna a week is the maximum allowed to keep within safe mercury levels)
- seaweed, this will decrease the bloat-potential of beans *and* increase your iodine consumption (killing two birds with one strip of seaweed!)
- pumpkin seeds and sunflower seeds.

A homemade nori roll with salmon and seeds or an oven-baked piece of salmon with a crunchy nut and seed coating are guaranteed to provide all the thyroid-stimulating nutrients in one juicy mouthful. A vegetarian option is the following scrumptious yoghurt dip that is nutritionally dense in tyrosine, iodine, zinc and selenium.

Dukkahish dip

1 cup organic yoghurt with acidophilus and bifidus

2 teaspoons kelp granules

¼ cup roughly chopped Brazil nuts

1 generous tablespoon lightly ground pumpkin seeds, dry roasted

1 generous tablespoon lightly ground sunflower seeds, dry roasted

1 teaspoon ground coriander seeds, toasted until fragrant

1 teaspoon ground cumin seeds, toasted until fragrant
sea salt to taste

Mix all ingredients together and plop a generous dollop on top of steamed or baked vegetables. Truly delicious with baked-root vegetables, a bowl of lentils or lima beans. Serve with crusty sourdough multi-seed bread.

Goitrogenic foods

Some foods when eaten in excess can suppress thyroid function, these include: brussels sprouts, broccoli, cauliflower, Chinese greens, cabbage spinach and turnip. These vegetables contain isothiocyanates that can block iodine absorption and should be eaten in moderation if you suspect a sluggish thyroid. However, in defence of the brassica family I must add that these vegetables also contain a photochemical that protects against some forms of cancer. By simply adding a good sprinkling of kelp granules to meals largely comprised of these vegetables, we can by-pass this iodine blockade.

HERBAL MEDICINE

There are a number of herbs that support thyroid function, and, more specifically, treat a sluggish thyroid. *Coleus forskohlii*, *Cnidium monnieri* and bladderwrack are all excellent choices to combat thyroid gland laziness.

Forskolin, the active constituent of *Coleus*, increases

the production of cyclic adenosine monophosphate (cAMP). Cylic AMP delivers vital messages within the cell, stimulating thyroid hormone production. Even at low concentrations cAMP is able to induce a significant T4 release, increasing cellular activity and our metabolic rate.

Osthol, a plant constituent isolated from *Cnidium monnieri,* increases thyroid hormone synthesis by interacting with the receptor for thyroid-releasing hormone (TRH). *Cnidium* improves the function of the pituitary-thyroid axis. That's a mouthful I know, but stay with me while I explain because the function of this axis is crucial to thyroid health. You may recall that TRH, stored in the hypothalamus of the brain, tells another hormone TSH to get with it and push those T3 and T4 hormones on their way. TSH lives in the pituitary gland, a tiny but immensely important part of the brain. Therefore, *Cnidium* enables efficient communication along the pituitary-thyroid axis. This is essential for a bubbling, healthy metabolic rate. *Cnidium,* like *Coleus,* also increases cAMP and therefore thyroid hormone production.

Bladderwrack (*Fucus vesiculosis*)* is a rich source of iodine, and should be incorporated in any tonic treating hypothyroidism or goiters. It is especially helpful where obesity is associated with thyroid trouble. In herbal texts it is described as 'thyroid stimulating and weight reducing'. In a clinical trial, obese participants taking bladder-wrack extract in addition to a controlled diet achieved a significantly greater average weight loss than those on a controlled diet.

It is best not to self-prescribe herbal medicine for thyroid health. Consult your naturopath or herbalist for advice.

Note: bladderwrack is not to be taken during pregnancy or lactation, and may interfere with thyroid replacement therapies.

SKIPPING MEALS LOWERS THE METABOLIC RATE

Ponder this fact for a moment. Starvation reduces the resting metabolic rate by as much as 40 per cent. Even a limited restriction of food intake, aimed at reducing body weight by only 10 per cent, decreases energy expenditure. Eating on the other hand, increases energy expenditure. So that naturopathic mantra of 'never skip breakfast' has some sound, scientific evidence behind it. The less we eat and the longer we leave between meals the more there is a compensatory slowing of our metabolic rate. Our bodies go into a semi-starvation mode, a mini-diabetic crisis, stubbornly holding on to fat reserves. A sensible approach indeed. After all, our body doesn't know when we will eat again, so it slows down and keeps some fat stores in reserve, 'just in case'.

Eating three moderately sized meals each day, with two small metabolic-stimulating snacks in between, will have our metabolic rate bubbling along nicely. I see many, many clients who are eating very little, yet cannot lose weight.

A sensible eating regime combined with *regular* exercise is the best way to prevent that frustrating meal-skipping-induced weight plateau.

Stress and our metabolic rate

Our adrenal glands respond to excessive stress by secreting additional amounts of the hormone cortisol. Prolonged elevated levels of cortisol destroys muscle tissue, increases body fat and interferes with magnesium absorption. And since even a mild magnesium deficiency predisposes us to stress, we can end up in a stress-induced cortisol–magnesium-deficient cycle. A magnesium deficiency also increases insulin resistance and the risk of developing mature onset diabetes.

Cortisol has been shown to induce leptin resistance. Leptin is a hormone that circulates in the blood at levels correlated to body-fat mass. It signals the brain to stop eating, to eat less or to burn calories faster (fish oils reduce leptin levels). So, prolonged stress ultimately results in a slower metabolic rate and an inability to accurately read signals of satiety between the gut and the brain. Not to mention the weight-gaining impact of using food as medication when depressed, stressed or anxious.

An enlightening study in 2002 illustrated the relationship between stress and weight gain. A total of 59 middle-aged men volunteered for stress and depression assessments using well-recognised measurement techniques – the Hamilton depression scale (HDS), the Beck depression inventory (BDI) and the Hamilton anxiety scale (HAS). The study showed that there was a direct relationship between symptoms of depression and stress and abdominal obesity. The higher the level of depression or stress, the greater the amount of stomach fat.

The hormone adrenalin, commonly referred to as our 'fight or flight' hormone, is secreted when we are under stress. Adrenalin stimulates the heart, increases blood pressure and heart rate, decreases blood flow to the digestive organs and, most importantly in respect of this discussion, raises blood-sugar levels and stimulates the liver to release more glucose and cholesterol into the blood. Not an ideal physiological state to be in at any time, but especially when attempting to lose weight. Sad to say, a lot of people remain in this heightened physiological state of stress for prolonged periods.

STRESS MANAGEMENT

Four nutrients are crucial to protecting against the toxic effects of stress: magnesium, vitamin C and vitamins B5 and B6. Magnesium lowers cortisol and insulin and enables muscles to uptake the amino acid creatine. Creatine boosts the growth of lean muscle tissue and improves the muscle's uptake of protein and water, leading to stronger muscles and a faster metabolic rate. Appropriate supplementation for prolonged stress would be: vitamin B5

200 mg, three times a day; vitamin B6 100 mg, twice a day; vitamin C 2000 mg, in small divided doses; plus magnesium orotate and magnesium aspartate 300 mg and 200 mg a day, respectively. Adequate essential fatty acids (EFAs) in the form of fish oil (EPA) 3000 mg daily or flaxseed oil 5 ml twice daily with food, should also be incorporated to protect against leptin resistance.

Herbal medicine for long-term stress should include a combination of the adrenal adaptogenic herbs: Siberian ginseng, withania and gota kola; as well as the restorative and soothing nervine relaxants and tonics: skullcap, oats seed, vervain and lime flowers.

Naturally, exercise has a bountiful benefit, as it increases our metabolic rate, tones our muscle tissue, improves bowel function, stimulates digestion *and* decreases stress and depression. Indeed, high-intensity exercise can be as effective as drugs in treating anxiety and depression, without any of the negative side effects. Every inch of our gastrointestinal tract benefits from regular, brisk exercise. Walking is perfect.

....

Christine's main health concern was a recent and inexplicable hair loss. She even brought with her to the consultation a small plastic bag containing evidence of her losses . . . it was significant. Being a brunette living in a newly renovated home of white and beige tones only reinforced the problem. Christine said that the bathroom floor and bedroom carpets needed to be mopped and vacuumed daily.

Christine also complained of a gradual but steady weight gain over the past year or so, even though little had changed in her reasonably healthy diet, and of feeling fatigued, especially in the mid-afternoon. She exercised regularly but rarely raised a sweat, and felt the cold intensely. Despite the warm, sunny day outside, Christine was wearing a jumper and looked cold – she was pale and displayed a curled-up body language. Christine noted that her bowels had always been sluggish. She rarely experienced a daily bowel motion, and was frequently uncomfortable and distended in the abdominal region.

Christine was 51 years of age, 165 cm tall and now weighed 65 kg. A year ago she weighed 58 kg, a weight she had maintained for the past 15 years with just the occasional minor fluctuation. She was the most charming woman, well-informed about diet and exercise and highly motivated. She ran a busy travel agency, employing 10 staff, which she clearly enjoyed but had found increasingly demanding in recent times.

Christine's nail analysis showed a possible zinc deficiency (white spots), a lack of digestive enzymes or hydrochloric acid (vertical lines) and a fairly conclusive thyroid dysfunction evidenced by transverse grooved, thin, splitting nails. Her nail beds were pale and, when light pressure was applied, failed to return to their normal colour quickly (poor circulation).

A discussion of Christine's diet revealed a few metabolic

hiccups. Despite knowing better, Christine had taken to skipping breakfast, due to increased demands on her time by her business. This often meant she was not eating anything until two in the afternoon. Lunch was either a large salad, with eggs or baked beans as the protein component, and for dinner she often steamed either broccoli, cauliflower or brussels sprouts (I had found a fellow brussel sprouts devotee at last!), plus eggplant, sweet potato, zucchini and tofu or lentils. Christine was a vegetarian who rarely ate dairy (not quite a vegan due to the egg factor), and admitted that she had, like most of us, become a creature of habit with her meals, especially the evening meal. She frequently arrived home late, not wanting to think about what to cook, and, on automatic pilot, put those same veggies in the steamer. Snacks included almonds and walnuts, soy yoghurt and the occasional sweet biscuit.

As you can see, Christine was certainly not overeating but she was consuming a fair amount of goitrogenic (foods that suppress thyroid function) vegetables. She was almost certainly low in iodine (no fish, seaweed etc.) and probably lacking in tyrosine, due to her dairy-free vegetarianism. I could almost guarantee she was low in zinc, too. And, as a fellow vegetarian, I say this with the greatest of respect: most vegetarians are zinc deficient due to a low intake of zinc-rich foods and a high intake of zinc-binding foods. The zinc taste test confirmed my suspicions. Christine's response was: 'Quite pleasant. It tastes just like water.' Not good.

Christine's blood pressure measured 98/66, indicating

slight hypotension. This would almost certainly account for Christine's poor circulation and sluggish metabolism, as well as her tendency to dizziness when standing up quickly. Low-blood pressure, dehydration and hunger are not good bedfellows – so frequent glasses of water and small frequent meals must be the order of the day.

*Christine had no objection to dairy. She had excluded it completely for several months to see if it helped with her bowel problems, and had just forgotten to reintroduce it. I therefore asked Christine to alternate soy yoghurt with cow or sheep's yoghurt, in order to increase her tyrosine intake, and to vary her vegetables, preferably **not** consuming the cabbage family on a daily basis. Also, breakfast became a non-negotiable 'must have' – either a bowl of porridge (low on the glycemic index) and a handful of ground pumpkin and sunflowers seeds (rich in zinc), or else 4 tablespoons of seed mix and an additional tablespoon of ground pumpkin seeds plus a good dollop of yoghurt. Five ml of flaxseed oil was to be stirred into breakfast and the same amount poured over one other meal of the day. This would provide a good balance of Omega 3 and Omega 6 EFAs, crucial to metabolism as well as to a healthy bowel and lustrous hair. Lunch needed to include a protein component: nuts, seeds, eggs or beans, and tofu was to be consumed no more than twice a week. A generous sprinkling of kelp granules was to be added to Christine's vegetables at dinner time. (See Appendix 15 for protein combinations for vegetarians.)*

To encourage circulation to her scalp I recommended Christine massage her scalp each night with a light tapping action using rolled-up fists. To stimulate hair follicles and encourage growth, I gave her a herbal oil to rub into the scalp and leave on overnight once a week.

Christine was commendably dedicated to her exercise routine. Although it was adequate, I felt she needed a new challenge and suggested that she start waking up some other muscle groups. She employed a personal trainer to construct a new exercise routine that included weights, kick-boxing and short sprints mixed with brisk arm-pumping walking. To her credit, she embraced her new routine with real vim.

I prescribed a supplement containing generous amounts of vitamins B5 and B6, and magnesium to support adrenal gland function and protect the nervous system; plus a formula containing iodine, tyrosine, chromium and zinc. Together these supplements would kick-start Christine's metabolic rate. I also gave Christine a liquid zinc drink to take 4 ml twice a day in 400 ml of water. Last, I gave this lovely client a diet diary in which to record every morsel of food entering her mouth, noting the time of day each meal or snack was consumed as well as the exercise undertaken. I suggested that Christine fax this diary back to me a few days before our next consultation, giving me time to go through it with a fine toothcomb.

I am very pleased to report that two weeks later Christine had already lost 2 kg and was actually eating more, her energy levels had increased dramatically and her bowel was also on *the mend – Christine was achieving a bowel motion almost daily. After a lifetime of infrequent motions this was a real breakthrough! Four weeks later her hair was looking decidedly thicker and she happily reported that there was no longer a trail of hairs across her bathroom floor. Within three months Christine had effortlessly managed to lose 10 kg and had a gorgeous head of thick, shiny hair to complement her new slimmer and, more importantly, healthier self.*

....

15

INFLAMMATORY BOWEL DISEASE

Inflammatory bowel disease (IBD) encompasses two debilitating and painful diseases of the bowel: ulcerative colitis and Crohn's disease. Although these two diseases have unique signs and symptoms, they do share a few characteristics. Both diseases are chronic, with periods of alternating relapse and remission. Diarrhoea is a common symptom. IBD can occur at any age; however, the most common age of onset is between 10 and 40. The disease can develop suddenly or have a gradual onset, and symptoms may be mild or very severe. There is some evidence to suggest that the severity of symptoms and relapse rates vary with the seasons, with the highest incidence in winter and autumn and the lowest incidence in summer.

There has been much speculation about the causes of IBD. Genetic predisposition (patients with IBD will usually have a close relative also suffering with either Crohn's disease or ulcerative colitis), immune disturbances, dietary factors, microbial infection, psychosomatic factors and vascular trauma have all been advanced as causative factors. However, the most outstanding contributing factor is undoubtedly diet. Patients with IBD almost invariably experience a flare-up when dietary guidelines are not followed. Smoking has also been suggested as a contributing factor in the occurence of IBD.

Drug therapy for both diseases normally involves sulphasalazine (a combination of a sulpha drug and aspirin) as well as steroids and salicylates, and broad spectrum antibiotics. Unfortunately these drugs deplete the body of iron, folic acid, vitamins C and D, potassium, zinc, magnesium and selenium. A double whammy, so to speak, since IBD generally reduces folic acid, iron, vitamin D and potassium levels.

Crohn's disease

All layers of the bowel wall are normally inflamed in Crohn's disease (also known as regional enteritis). The ileum and cecum are the most commonly affected sites, although any part of the large and small intestine can be affected. Crohn's disease is characterised by intermittent bouts of non-bloody diarrhoea and a low-grade fever. Many sufferers may have no specific symptoms for years other than an 'irritable' bowel. The hallmark symptom of Crohn's disease is recurrent episodes of pain in the lower-right part of the abdomen or above the pubic bone, which is often preceded or alleviated by defecation. An abdominal or pelvic mass is often visible; bloating, nausea and vomiting may also occur. Fistulas (narrow channels) may form in the perianal region between the loops of the intestine or even extend into the bladder. Anaemia resulting from malabsorption of vitamin B12 is common, and folic acid and vitamin D deficiency may also occur. X-rays show abnormality of the terminal ileum. In Crohn's disease constipation normally only occurs as a symptom of obstruction in the small intestine.

Foods that have been implicated in Crohn's disease include:

- refined sugar
- carrageenan (carrageenan is an extract from red seaweeds and used by the food industry to stabilise milk products; in particular chocolate, cottage cheese, ice-cream and flavoured milks)
- shellfish
- yeast
- sweeteners
- fats
- corn
- wheat, particularly wheat bran.

Food allergies will also increase inflammation, exacerbating Crohn's disease, and may be a causative factor in predisposed individuals.

Ulcerative colitis

The large intestine and rectum are the areas of the GIT most affected in ulcerative colitis. Frequent diarrhoea with small amounts of blood and purulent mucus is extremely common. In some cases of ulcerative colitis, diarrhoea can be so severe that up to 30–40 bowel motions can be experienced each day. Indeed, I had one poor patient a few years ago, whose life was ruled by her bowel. She was able to leave the house for only short periods of time, and then to areas where she knew there were public toilets.

Ulcers, haemorrhoids and fistulas are nearly always found around the anal passage. Pain is not a prominent symptom of ulcerative colitis, but severe pain can occur during flare-ups, and a vague discomfort in the lower abdomen or cramps in the mid-section of the abdomen can occur at any time. Constipation occurs very occasionally, and this is when the inflamed rectum triggers a reflex response in the colon that causes it to retain the stool. Weight loss, fever, dehydration and anaemia are caused by fluid loss, bleeding and inflammation. Diagnosis is usually confirmed by X-ray or sigmoidoscopy (an internal examination of the colon). Ulcerative colitis is associated with an increased risk of colon cancer.

Dietary factors that have been implicated in ulcerative colitis include:
- wheat
- dairy

- caffeine
- spicy foods
- fatty meats.

Food allergies must be eliminated as they increase inflammation of the bowel, thus exacerbating ulcerative colitis.

Treatment for Crohn's disease and ulcerative colitis

Generally speaking, treatment for both diseases focuses on: quelling inflammation, healing intestinal mucosas, decreasing free-radical damage, reversing nutritional deficiencies and eliminating causative factors. Our naturopathic tools, therefore, include: Omega 3 fatty acids, bioflavonoids, glutamine, slippery elm and probiotics; as well as herbs such as: meadowsweet, golden seal, chamomile, astragalus and echinacea. The anti-oxidant nutrients include: vitamins A, C and E, and the minerals zinc and selenium. And dietary changes are always a crucial part of preventing or limiting the re-occurrence of IBDs.

....

Julian was 22 when he came to see me after having spent 10 days in hospital following a debilitating flare-up of his Crohn's disease. He had been diagnosed with Crohn's six months prior to our appointment and had not yet rearranged his diet to try to increase the remission time and decrease the relapses. Julian managed a bistro and a nightclub as well as studying financial planning part-time. He was a charming young man with a lot on his plate.

Julian was taking a rather hefty dose of corticosteroids following his hospitalisation, which was to be gradually reduced over the course of the next few weeks. Julian's bowel had settled down, but he was now suffering from constipation as a result of the medication in hospital. I asked Julian about his diet. A typical daily menu looked like this: breakfast was Corn Flakes with milk, or toast and Vegemite. Lunch was either a cooked meal of meat and vegetables or a cheese-and-ham toasted sandwich on white bread. He frequently had takeaway for dinner, with pizza and curries being favourites, and he drank beer four nights out of seven, with a rather large over-indulgence on Friday or Saturday night. Since the recent flare-up, however, Julian had not touched a drop of alcohol.

I immediately adjusted Julian's diet to exclude all dairy products, yeast-containing foods and alcohol. Corn Flakes were similarly banished. I suggested that he start his day with a bowel of cooked whole oats moistened with oat milk or rice milk; have a multigrain or rye sourdough salad sandwich with salmon or chicken for lunch (Julian was not too enthusiastic about exploring vegetarian options); and for dinner have cooked vegetables and protein, with either Basmati or brown rice, or rice or buckwheat pasta. I also asked him to eat plenty of fruit, especially bananas and papaya, and to drink 2 L of water every day.

The ileum is commonly affected in Crohn's disease, so I assumed that Julian's vitamin B12 levels were poor because vitamin B12 is absorbed in this part of the intestine. Similarly, his folic acid levels would have been compromised by the administration of the steroid medication; unfortunately, a folic acid deficiency causes further malabsorption due to the altered structure of the cells of the intestinal mucosa. These cells have a very rapid turnover (changing every one to four days) and need a constant supply of folic acid. Luckily, Julian's blood-test results did not show anaemia, although his iron and ferritin levels were **just** within the reference range. I prescribed a supplement containing folic acid, vitamin B12 and slippery elm. The mucilaginous quality of slippery elm soothes, protects and heals the gastric mucosa and promotes absorption of the other nutrients. I also prescribed zinc picolinate 15 mg, three times a day, to help heal the intestinal mucosa, and a vitamin C supplement with a strong component of bioflavonoids; namely quercitin and hesperidin to quell inflammation and prevent fistula formation.

The bistro Julian manages had a juicer, so I asked him to prepare a glass of cabbage juice and sip slowly prior to lunch. Cabbage juice contains substance 'U', which is superbly effective at healing ulceration, and it is actually quite pleasant, having a mild salty taste and almost effervescent consistency. A probiotic supplement was also prescribed to replenish the friendly bacteria that had been destroyed by antibiotics and to help re-establish vitamin B12 levels, to be taken twice daily on an empty stomach. Lactobacillus and bifidus, two of the five strains in the formula, would also help restore normal bowel motions. (The authors of the large-scale study of the human colon genome referred to on page 55, suggest that altering the microbe population in the gut may be an effective treatment for IBD, as well as reducing food allergies and obesity.) For Julian's mild anal fissures, I suggested he locally apply either aloe vera gel or paw paw ointment to accelerate the healing process of this delicate tissue.

Julian was extremely compliant. The shock of his recent hospitalisation had, I think, reinforced the seriousness of the disease and the importance of lifestyle and diet in stabilising his condition. Within two weeks Julian's bowel was back on track with one to two well-formed bowel motions per day, without pain or urgency. His skin tone was much improved with colour returning to his cheeks, and his energy levels had gone up a notch. I checked Julian's zinc levels with the taste-perception test, and there was a slight improvement. I had not expected a rapid improvement because Julian's bowel was undergoing major repair, and his immune system had been severely compromised. So he maintained the three-a-day regime until the next appointment. Two weeks later, Julian passed the zinc taste test with flying colours, so I changed the zinc supplement to a strong anti-oxidant containing therapeutic levels of zinc, selenium, vitamins A, C and E as well as the B group vitamins. I also swapped the folic acid, B12 and slippery elm supplement for a powder containing glutamine,

slippery elm, apple pectin and quercitin, which would
soothe and heal Julian's gastrointestinal tract. One generous
teaspoon of this powder to be taken twice daily before meals.
The probiotic powder could also be mixed into this to simplify
the supplementation regime.

Julian remained on this protocol for a further six weeks.
In the past two years he has had only one major flare-up, and
no return visits to the hospital. This hiccup in Julian's remission
was, in his own words, preceded by a 'big night out with the
boys', which involved copious amounts of alcohol and fatty
foods. I am pleased to report that in recent months Julian has
not touched a drop of alcohol and his diet is exemplary.

....

16

PEPTIC MATTERS: DUODENAL AND GASTRIC ULCERS

While inflammatory bowel disease (IBD) usually involves ulceration of the bowel walls, a peptic ulcer is an ulcerative disorder of the upper-gastrointestinal tract (GIT), where the wall lining and the tissues beneath have been eroded, leaving an open wound. This may be caused by an excess of stomach acid, insufficient production of mucus to protect the stomach lining, or both. There are two common types of ulcers: duodenal and gastric; the difference between the two ulcers is their location. The duodenal ulcer occurs, naturally enough, in the duodenum, the narrow section of the small intestine connecting it to the stomach; while the gastric ulcer's preferred site of irritation is the main part of the stomach.

Symptoms of a peptic ulcer

A burning, gnawing pain located somewhere between the breastbone and navel is often the first symptom of a peptic ulcer, and is frequently accompanied by heartburn, nausea, loss of appetite and indigestion. The usual onset of pain is 45–60 minutes after a meal. Pain may vary from moderate to severe, and may wake up the sufferer during the night. Other symptoms can include: lower back pain, headache, a choking sensation, vomiting and blood in the stool. Diagnosis is normally confirmed by an X-ray or a fibre-optic examination.

Causes of a peptic ulcer

There are many factors that cause a peptic ulcer:

- Certain drugs, namely aspirin and non-steroidal anti-inflammatory drugs (NSAIDs). Taken over a long period of time, these drugs can wear away the lining of the digestive tract, causing bleeding and ulceration. Steroids, such as those taken for arthritis can also cause ulceration.
- Smoking wears away the stomach lining and bile-salt reflux induced by smoking is extremely irritating to the stomach.
- Calcium carbonate antacids can actually increase gastric acid secretion (the sodium bicarbonate type is believed to interfere with heart and kidney function).
- Stress and anxiety cause an increase in stomach acid.
- Bacteria, namely *Helicobacter pylori* (a breath test will confirm its presence), is believed to be

responsible for up to 90 per cent of gastric ulcers and 70 per cent of duodenal ulcers.
- Excessive vitamin C supplementation.
- Food sensitivities can cause inflammation that erodes the stomach lining. (I always put my clients whose blood tests reveal multiple food allergies on a course of the amino acid glutamine to heal their, undoubtedly, eroded lining.)

Treatment of a peptic ulcer

One of my first patients, who I treated at my naturopathic college's student clinic, presented with the classic signs of a peptic ulcer: a burning, gnawing pain in the stomach that commenced soon after eating. Relieved to have made such a quick diagnosis, I recommended a strong cup of chamomile tea each day and then roll around the floor immediately afterwards. Needless to say, this patient did not return for a follow-up consultation! While, as we shall see, this 'rolling herbal tea' method would have helped, there are far more effective and less physically demanding treatments for this painful condition of the upper GIT!

- Licorice root heals gastric and duodenal ulcers and should be the herb of choice for all ulcer sufferers. Take 750–1500 mg of deglycyrrhizinised licorice three times a day between meals for up to three months. Unlike drugs, which inhibit the release of acid, licorice increases the number of mucus-secreting cells therefore enhancing the protective lining of the GIT. All licorice addicts, please note, this does *not* mean increasing your consumption of licorice sweets. The herb is rarely found in a licorice stick!

- Raw cabbage juice contains high levels of glutamine and can potentially heal an ulcer within 14 days. Recent research suggests that cabbage also contains a phyto-nutrient capable of destroying *H. pylori*. Take 400–500 ml twice a day before meals. Make enough for each day and keep refrigerated. (Broccoli sprouts, which look like large snow pea sprouts, have been found to contain the same stomach-protecting phytonutrient as cabbage, which reduces the *H. pylori* bacteria as well as protecting against stomach cancer. Both vegetables are from the brassica family.)

- Slippery elm powder coats, soothes and heals gastric mucosa. Mix one tablespoon of slippery elm bark with a little purified water, then slowly add more water until the mixture resembles a thick milk shake. Drink twice a day between meals.

- Aloe vera juice – we are all familiar with the healing ability of aloe vera gel on an open cut or burn. The juice extract has a similar restorative effect on intestinal mucosa. Take 1/3 cup twice a

day on an empty stomach. Be sure to use a good-
quality whole-leaf extract.

- Glutamine is an amino acid with a special affinity
  for intestinal mucosa. It is the primary source of
  fuel for cells that line the stomach and intestine,
  and heals inflamed and ulcerated tissues. Take
  2000 mg three times a day on an empty stomach.
- Zinc heals gastric mucosa, stabilising many
  proteins and cell membranes. Steroid medication
  decreases zinc absorption. Use zinc carnosine to
  inhibit *Helicobacter pylori*, 12 mg twice a day;
  or if *H. pylori* is not a contributing factor use
  liquid zinc sulphate, 4 ml in 400 ml water twice
  a day after meals. Do *not* take zinc for longer
  than six weeks at this dose as it interferes with
  copper absorption. Ask your naturopath to check
  your zinc levels with a zinc taste-perception test
  regularly. Do *not* take zinc at the same time as
  iron, as iron deceases zinc absorption.
- Bioflavonoids, part of the vitamin C complex
  (rutin, hesperidin, quercitin and genistein), have
  anti-inflammatory, anti-histamine and anti-viral
  properties. Several of the flavanoids can inhibit *H.
  pylori* and prevent ulcer formation. Take 1000 mg
  twice a day with meals.
- Anti-oxidant supplementation with hefty amounts
  of zinc, selenium and vitamin E for healing.

- Essential fatty acids (EFAs) have a profound effect on the inflammatory process. They blunt the inflammatory response to endotoxins and ameliorate intestinal mucosal damage. The outer membrane that protects every cell in our body requires EFAs on a daily basis to form healthy, flexible, tightly sealed cell walls. Supplement with 5 ml of flaxseed oil twice a day with food; or take a combined evening primrose oil (EPO) and fish oil capsule, 1000 mg three times a day with meals.

- Eliminate food allergies. Either keep a diet diary for a week, recording every morsel that enters your mouth and associated symptoms, or have a blood test to determine the presence of IgG antibodies (your naturopath can provide a referral).

- Eliminate common irritants (not necessarily allergens), such as milk, alcohol, coffee, spicy foods, chocolate and citrus fruits. Consume small meals, frequently.

- Avoid cow's milk – it may neutralise stomach acid, but ultimately it worsens the condition because calcium and protein stimulate the production of more acid.

- Probiotics. If taking a course of antibiotic treatment for *H. pylori*, be sure to supplement with probiotics. This will replenish the beneficial intestinal flora that have been wiped out by the drug therapy. The way to get the most from your supplement is to take it on an empty stomach, preferably in a capsule with an enteric coating to protect it against the acidic stomach and intestinal secretions, and regularly – *not* the stop-and-start 'I forgot to take my supplement' approach. Choose a supplement that has at least 25 billion organisms (check the label), take one capsule twice a day.

- Eat plenty of green leafy vegetables. They are a good source of folic acid and vitamin K that are required for healing.

- Befriend bananas – these wonderful fruits contain a substance that stimulates the growth of mucosal cells that form a protective barrier of the stomach and intestines.

- Chamomile tea. Don't laugh, the old chamomile-tea-roll-around-the-floor method has a sound scientific rationale behind it. Chamomile is an anti-inflammatory herb, and a gentle nervous system relaxant effective in treating gut spasm and ulceration. Prepare a very strong cup of chamomile tea (i.e., use at least 2 heaped teaspoons of flowers per cup, preferably organic) and drink at room temperature. Gently roll from side to side to ensure the entire stomach lining is in contact with this magnificent herb. Drink and roll at least twice a day.

- Nervine herbs, such as verbena, chamomile, lemon balm and skullcap have a wonderfully relaxing action on the nervous system and soothe frayed nerves. It is important to de-stress.
- For periods of prolonged stress, the adaptogenic group of herbs has no rival! These herbs include Siberian ginseng, panax ginseng, withania, and gota kola. Their protective and restorative characteristics increase our resistance to stress.
- Introduce stress management techniques such as meditation, or similar relaxation practices, as well as a form of exercise that *you* enjoy.
- Meadowsweet (*Filipendula ulmaria*) is my favourite digestive remedy. It soothes and protects the mucous membranes of the GIT, reduces stomach acidity, eases nausea and contains compounds that help heal and prevent ulcers. Meadowsweet also contains salicylic acid, which reduces pain and inflammation of peptic ulceration (see Appendix 9).
- Marshmallow (*Althea officinalis*) – the leaves, roots and flowers of this beautiful herb contain polysaccharides which form a soothing gel that reduces stomach acidity, relieves heartburn and forms a protective coating that heals areas of inflammation along the digestive tract. (Please note aerated sugary pink and white puffs of

confectionary known as marshmallows are *not* therapeutic!)

- Golden seal (*Hydrastis canadensis*) is anti-microbial, anti-inflammatory, anti-haemorrhagic and restorative to fragile membrane, making it a superlative ulcer remedy. The traditional use of this herb has been for mucous membrane inflammation, peptic ulcer, dyspepsia and colitis, as well as a plethora of skin conditions – which probably goes a long way to explaining its now endangered existence. (As herbalists, we try to only ever include this herb in our remedies when there is absolutely no equally effective substitute.) Precaution: do *not* take golden seal during pregnancy or lactation.

    Golden seal is a particularly bitter and astringent herb (as is calendula, while on the topic of taste), so I generally advise my clients taking herbal medicine containing this herb, to dilute the 5 ml dose with about 10 ml water or fruit juice. (Diluting with cabbage juice would perhaps be pushing my naturopathic luck and patient compliance!) Swallow quickly in one go to reduce the contact time with taste buds. For very sensitive individuals, I suggest sucking on some ice beforehand to deaden the taste buds and the olfactory nerve or chill the entire bottle of herbs by storing in the fridge. (See Appendix 16, How to make that (herbal) medicine go down!)

- Echinacea (*Echinacea augustifolia/Echinacea purpurea*) is our most valuable immune-stimulating herb. It is used to treat bacterial, viral and fungal infections of the skin and mucous membranes, and treats external septic sores and abrasions. To assess the quality of your echinacea supplement, look for a tongue-tingling sensation caused by the main active constituent, alkylamides.

- Calendula (*Calendula officinalis*) contains anti-inflammatory and astringent properties. We all know how effective calendula ointment can be for local burns and slow-to-heal wounds; used internally this herb is as efficacious in healing ulcerated mucous membrane. Calendula is classified by herbalists as a cholagogue, that is, it encourages the discharge of bile into the duodenum, which alleviates indigestion and general gastrointestinal complaints. Precaution: do *not* take if you have a sensitivity to the compositae plant family; that is, ragweed, chrysanthemums and daisies.

Anti-ulcer herbal tonic

An example of a typical anti-ulcer herbal tonic I would put together in the clinic looks like this:

25 ml marshmallow root

30 ml echinacea
15 ml calendula*
30 ml meadowsweet

Take 5 ml three times a day with meals.

*Hydrastis could be substituted for calendula in especially acute or complex cases.

Anti-ulcer juice

This is a simple remedy you can prepare at home that soothes any irritated surfaces of the upper GIT. Be sure to sip slowly and try to 'chew' your juice.

½ bunch silverbeet
2 carrots
½ head cabbage
handful broccoli sprouts
30 ml aloe vera juice
1 teaspoon slippery elm powder (optional)

Cut the cabbage into wedges and feed through a juicer, followed by the silverbeet (wrap in a large cabbage leaf for easy juicing) and then the carrots. Mix 400 ml of the fresh juice with 30 ml good-quality aloe vera juice and sip slowly twice a day before meals. For added healing benefits, mix one teaspoon slippery elm powder to a paste with a little purified water and stir into the juice.

17

HEALTHY GUT GUIDE SOLUTIONS

At last we are here, committed to reorganising our diets to overcome our individual digestive disorders! We can pull our newly acquired knowledge and must-dos into a *workable* and *enjoyable* eating plan – something that can be applied every day without too much angst-provoking, time-consuming preparation. However, bear in mind that being in control of what we place in our mouths is essential to healing our gut complaints; non-self-prepared options are never going to be as beneficial.

Creating a balanced, healthy lifestyle in order to achieve a pain-free gut *does* take some effort. If we do not have time in the evening to prepare a gut-friendly, nutritious evening meal as well as lunch for the next day, then it will take just 60 minutes on the weekend to pre-prepare meals for the week: grate and/or chop vegetables for lunches and evening meals, cook and freeze legumes and pulses, make a large pot of soup, pre-cook brown rice. This forethought and preparation will guide us painlessly through our busy working weeks. Aim at your goal with undivided attention and enthusiasm. You *can* do it. It just requires focus, determination and enthusiasm! And the rewards far outweigh the effort.

All the elements required for a pain-free gastrointestinal tract (GIT) are covered in this chapter. Let's see how effortlessly these natural solutions translate into our everyday dietary choices.

Daily dietary essentials

- adequate and appropriate fibre; at least 50 g a day; increase fibre intake slowly, favouring soluble fibre
- minimum of 2 L water
- enzyme-rich fresh, seasonal foods
- prebiotic and probiotic rich foods
- essential fatty acids (EFAs), a balanced range of Omega 3 and Omega 6
- sound food combinations; no fruit and animal proteins and *no* double proteins
- a variety of grains; eliminate wheat for six weeks and choose gluten-free grains
- keep spices and other gut irritants to an absolute minimum
- keep stimulants to an absolute minimum (caffeine, alcohol, sugar)
- reduce intake of sulphur-containing foods

• eliminate cow's milk if lactose intolerant, otherwise keep dairy to a minimum – yoghurt excepted.

Bear in mind personal idiosyncracies. For example, if a high-fructose diet causes discomfort, then snack on plums or kiwifruit rather than pears; or, if you are gluten intolerant, favour rice or buckwheat porridge instead of muesli. Make it *work* for you. To treat specific bowel concerns see the relevant chapter for additional guidelines.

Eating technique

The only non-dietary items you need to add to the above guidelines are a relaxed environment and a good chewing technique – in other words, no gulping down meals in a hurried, anxious manner. Follow these tips to guarantee a pain-free GIT:

• chew each mouthful thoughtfully and thoroughly
• never overeat; stop before you are too full
• never eat when anxious, upset or angry
• do not hurry meals; slow down your eating.

Healthy Gut Guide diet options

BREAKFAST

• always drink a glass of warm water and fresh lemon juice on rising, followed by a brisk 45-minute walk or equivalent exercise

- whole barley flakes or oats, cooked or soaked overnight with stewed apples and chopped walnuts
- homemade muesli
- buckwheat porridge and baked plums
- cooked brown rice with banana and raisins
- oat bran or barley bran porridge
- brown rice cakes with tahini and avocado.

Tip: add either apple or pear juice, soy milk, rice milk or oat milk to moisten grain cereals; plus seed mix for extra fibre and flaxseed oil for EFAs.

LUNCH

- homemade soups, add beans or lentils to thicken
- stir-fried vegetables and tofu with tamari sauce
- steamed veggies (cold) with tuna, salmon or lentils
- mountain bread wraps (come in a wonderful variety of rice, oat or barley grain), filled with grated beetroot, carrots, alfalfa sprouts, spinach leaves, cooked sweet potato and tahini
- brown rice or buckwheat kernel salads with a selection of vegetables plus either chicken, omelet, kidney beans or chickpeas
- generous salad of beetroot, carrot, rocket, raddicchio, sprouts, celeriac and baby spinach, plus either salmon, egg, chickpeas, lentils or a handful of almonds or walnuts

- toasted rye sourdough or seed-bread sandwich with the above salad (or as much as you can squash between those slices of bread), plus either hummus, eggs, salmon or tofu and avocado.

DINNER

- baked root vegetables with hummus and avocado dressing
- vegetable casseroles, including corn, beans, potato with the skin, broccoli, and cauliflower and whole baby carrots served on basmati rice
- steamed or stir-fried vegetables (use olive oil), including a good selection of brassica family vegetables (broccoli, brussels sprouts, cauliflower); orange and red vegetables (sweet potato, carrot, red cabbage, pumpkin); plus green leaves (spinach, Chinese broccoli, silverbeet), and a protein component of either fish, organic chicken, tofu, tempeh or legumes. Sprinkle with 5 ml flaxseed oil. If desired, a complex carbohydrate can also be added, such as brown rice, buckwheat or spelt pasta, polenta and quinoa.
- omelets with salad
- goat's cheese feta sprinkled over steamed vegetables and baked beetroot with wild rice
- fish, organic chicken or tofu marinated in tamari and fresh herbs, with sliced eggplant, tomato,

corn and potato with skin, all grilled on the
barbeque with large green salad
- crispy tempeh and avocado and tahini dip (see
  Appendix 5).

Tip: add a teaspoon of kelp granules to your dinner plate
at least once a week for a healthy thyroid gland; sip a glass
of water with a teaspoon of apple cider vinegar with dinner if digestion is especially poor.

DESSERT

- baked fruit: apples, peaches or pears stuffed with
  chopped figs
- stewed plums or apricots
- fresh dates, just a few
- homemade yoghurt and blueberries
- mixed berries: blackberries, raspberries,
  strawberries.

SNACKS

- fresh fruit in season: try to vary every day but *no*
  melons, pineapple or grapes
- nuts and seeds in moderation: a small handful
  almonds or walnuts; 3–4 Brazil nuts; a small
  handful sunflower and pumpkin seeds, chewed well
- yoghurts: sheep's milk, goat's milk, cow's milk
  or soy. Choose according to your own digestive
  capacity but vary as much as possible. Or even

better, make your own with the best-quality
soy or rice milk you can find (see Appendix 6,
Homemade yoghurt).
- rice cakes with almond spread, avocado or
mashed banana
- buckwheat crisp breads with above toppings
- vegetable juices: carrot, beetroot, celery or
parsley. Sip very slowly. Juices should be 'chewed'
not gulped. Imagine consuming the equivalent
amount of vegetables in the time it takes to gulp
your juice. Not comfortable!

WATER

Drink 2 L a day – not negotiable!

HERBAL TEAS

Vary your herbal teas, include each of the following weekly:
- meadowsweet
- dandelion
- chamomile
- peppermint
- ginger.

Getting the portion size right

Generally I don't like my clients to worry too much about
the amount of food they eat at each meal. Food choices are
far more important than portion sizes. Indeed, studies

have shown that most people, on average, eat a very similar amount of food. However, I do recognise that it is often helpful to have a few guidelines when embarking on a health regime. Just so there can be no confusion, here are a few portion size hints. I must admit my lack of size direction once resulted in a client returning for a follow-up visit complaining of extreme hunger shortly after eating breakfast. To my horror I discovered she was only eating 4 *teaspoons* of seed mix for breakfast instead of the desired 4 *tablespoons*! I should have been a lot clearer in my directions.

THE PALM METHOD

No measuring cups, spoons, bowls or scales needed, just a hand minus the thumb and fingers – figuratively speaking, that is. This measure will give the approximate amount of protein (fish, chicken, tofu, eggs) that should be consumed per meal. Likewise, the same palm measurement is used to estimate the amount of carbohydrate to be consumed; except in the carbohydrate case, it is two palms of complex carbohydrates per meal (steamed vegetables, oats, fruit salad).

For legumes and beans, which can be classified as carbohydrates or (incomplete) proteins, use one and a half palms. The amount of EFAs eaten each day should range from 10–30 ml. This would roughly equate to one metric teaspoon of flaxseed oil twice a day plus a small handful of nuts or a thick slice of avocado.

Extra tips for digestive happiness

- Eat according to the seasons and vary your diet as much as possible.
- Check your evening meal for colour – green, orange, red and yellow should all be present.
- Think of a vegetable or fruit you haven't eaten for a while and incorporate it in next week's meals.
- Keep meals clean: not too many spices, dressings, or mixing of proteins. The most nutritious and delicious meals are often the simplest: the splendour of a fresh bowl of figs, a salad of homegrown tomatoes, basil and cucumber (peeled) with a little sea salt, a slice of rye sourdough spread with avocado and tahini. Eating food as close to the way nature provided is best.
- Prepare your meals from scratch.
- Avoid packaged or processed foods containing a multitude of additives and preservatives.

Pain-free gut protocol

The following is a general guide to ensure sound GIT health and to resolve any minor gut issues. See relevant chapters for specific measures. If you are under additional stress it may be necessary to increase your B vitamins, magnesium and vitamin C, and consider some adaptogenic herbs such as Siberian ginseng, withania, gota kola, plus some sooth-ing nervines, principally oats seed, lime flowers, vervain

and skullcap. It is always advised to consult your naturopath or herbalist because appropriate dosages and blends
are vital in obtaining a therapeutic result.

SUPPLEMENTS

Follow these recommendations, for a minimum of six
weeks and up to three months.

- Aloe vera juice (whole-leaf extract) heals the entire
  GIT and softens stools. Take ¼ cup twice a day
  before meals.
- Glutamine heals a porous intestinal lining and
  ulceration. Take 2000 mg twice a day before meals.
- Vitamin B complex protects the central nervous
  system and the enteric nervous system and
  promotes the manufacture of bowel flora. Choose a
  supplement that contains at least 50 mg each of the
  B group vitamins; except folic acid and B12 which
  should be a minimum of 400 mcg and 100 mcg,
  respectively. Take once a day after breakfast.
- Magnesium decreases reactions to food allergies,
  relaxes the gut musculature and ensures
  efficient insulin uptake. Take a daily supplement
  containing 300 mg magnesium orotate and
  200 mg magnesium aspartate.
- Plant-derived pancreatic enzymes break down
  fats, carbohydrates and protein. Take one capsule
  15 minutes before each meal.

- Probiotics reintroduce bowel flora in the small and large intestine. Take a supplement containing a minimum of 25 billion *Lactobacillus acidophilus* and *Bifidobacterium lactis*, twice a day before meals (keep refrigerated).
- For a sluggish metabolism add 200 mcg chromium amino acid chelate or chromium nicotinate, incorporated in a glucose tolerance factor (GTF) formula, three times a day.

HERBAL MEDICINE

To soothe an uncomfortable gut and ensure good bowel health consider the following herbs (best prescribed by a qualified naturopath).

- St Mary's thistle (*Silybum marianum*) – a gentle liver tonic capable of regenerating liver cells.
- Lime flowers (*Tilia europea*) – an anti-spasmodic, especially effective for gut pain as well as migraine.
- Vervain (*Verbena officinalis*) – combines the actions of a nervine tonic, anti-spasmodic and a liver tonic. An excellent combination for GIT problems related to a sluggish liver.
- Cramp bark (*Virburnum opulus*) – one of our best anti-spasmodic herbs, a superb relaxer of muscular and visceral tension.
- Dandelion root (*Taraxacum officinalis*) – the root of

this under-appreciated herb is effective for liver and gallbladder disorders. It is part of every herbalist's repertoire for sluggish bowels and constipation.

- Meadowsweet (*Filipendula ulmaria*) – an antacid, as well as possessing anti-inflammatory actions. Meadowsweet is one of the best digestive remedies: reducing acidity, easing nausea and healing mucous membranes.
- Fringe tree (*Chionanthus virginicus*) – one of my favourite herbs, this delightful herb can be used for liver problems, gallbladder inflammation and also acts as a gentle diuretic and laxative.
- Chamomile (*Matricaria recutita*) – an anti-spasmodic, heals inflamed gastric mucosa, soothes the nervous system and encourages bile release. (What more could a herbalist wish for!)

HEALTHY GUT GUIDE TO HERBAL TEAS

These herbal tea remedies can be drunk hot or cold, or with a slice of lemon or lime.

For abdominal pain and bloating

These gentle carminative herbs are excellent for relaxing spasm and bloating in the gut, and for releasing trapped wind and gas. Indeed, in naturopathic circles chamomile is sometimes called 'the mother of the gut', referring to its ability to relieve pain and tenderness and promote digestion and relaxation. Chamomile is also anti-microbial (fights infection in the digestive system) and stimulates the formation of new tissue in eroded areas of the lining of the GIT.

Mix together equal portions of the following herbs. Always try to obtain organic dried herbs where possible.

meadowsweet
peppermint
chamomile*
fennel

Add two generous teaspoons to a plunger and wait 10 minutes before straining and drinking. For an added therapeutic effect, add a whole cinnamon quill (anti-microbial and anti-spasmodic) just before drinking and serve in your favourite bone china cup. (The therapeutic effect of visual beauty and touch perceptions cannot be underestimated.) And a silent word of thanks to the herbal kingdom for its generosity and kindness wouldn't go astray either.

*Note: chamomile is known to have an adverse response in people allergic to the daisy family (compositae or asteraceae).

For sluggish digestion and liver

This herbal blend is quite bitter and, therefore, an excellent liver stimulant, and the fringe tree, through its action of releasing bile, is especially therapeutic for a sluggish bowel.

1 teaspoon dandelion root
½ teaspoon globe artichoke*
1 teaspoon St Mary's thistle
½ teaspoon fringe tree bark

Place herbs into a warmed china or glass teapot and add 2 cups boiling water. Leave to steep for 10 minutes before straining. Drink 1–2 cups a day.

Note: globe artichoke should be used with caution by those who have liver cancer, liver disease (cirrhosis) or bile-duct obstruction, and it may have an adverse response in people allergic to the daisy family (compositae or asteraceae).

LIFESTYLE – DAILY ROUTINES AND GOOD HABITS

Healthy gastrointestinal wellbeing is obtained and maintained by an intelligent lifestyle.

- Remember, good bowel habits are aquired. Our bowel can be taught new tricks! Raise those feet off the lavatory floor – squatting can be achieved with a mininum of fuss, and dignity need not be compromised.

- Exercise is crucial to good bowel health: brisk walking, yoga, Pilates and a hearty belly laugh are all GIT-friendly activities. Brisk whole-body, dry-skin brushing (use a rough towel or loofah if a body brush is unavailable) before showering each morning, is an invigorating way to kick-start your day.

- Relax: let go of tension in the stomach and bowel, consciously relax the abdominal muscles. Leave a note to remind yourself, in the car or on your desk, until it becomes second nature to unwind and unknot.
- Cultivate calmness: concentrate on letting go. Practising gratitude helps.

APPENDIX : 1

. . . .

THE ROLE OF ENZYMES IN DIGESTION

The small intestinal enzymes lactase, maltase and sucrase, plus the pancreatic enzymes amylase, protease and lipase break down the food we eat into nutrients that are able to be absorbed and utilised by the body.

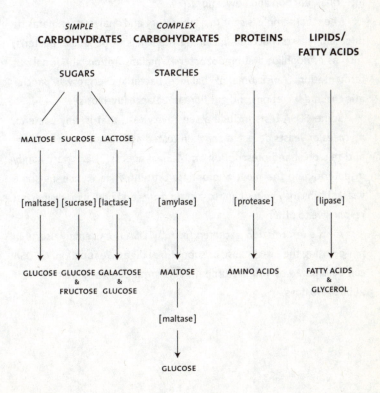

APPENDIX 2

COMPLETE DIGESTIVE STOOL ANALYSIS (CDSA)

This invaluable test accurately determines exactly what is going on in your large and small intestine. The CDSA test involves the collection of a stool specimen in the privacy of your own bathroom, on either one or three consecutive days (depending on the level of analysis required). It provides an overview of all the components of digestion, absorption, intestinal function and bowel flora.

The stool sample is sent to a laboratory and analysed for: parasitic infection, yeasts, bacteria (including the levels of beneficial bacteria, such as acidophilus and bifidobacteria), malabsorption, abnormal gut fermentation, transit time, pH balance, bacterial overgrowth, pancreatic enzyme secretions and gut flora imbalance (dysbiosis).

Some CDSA tests include a sensitivity test, that is, any bacteria, mycoses or yeasts detected are then tested against a panel of natural anti-microbial and prescription anti-fungal agents. This is very handy in determining the most appropriate anti-infective to use, as some yeast strains may be resilient to certain drugs and herbal medicine, but responsive to others.

All the information gathered from a CDSA is extremely useful in pin-pointing the exact cause of suboptimal digestive function. A CDSA can be ordered by your naturopath and turnaround time for results is about 7–10 days.

APPENDIX : 3

SEED MIX

> 250 mg golden linseeds
> 250 mg sesame seeds
> 250 mg sunflower seeds
> 250 mg pumpkin seeds
> 1 kg fine oat bran, barley bran or rice bran

Grind the seeds in a blender, mix the ground seeds with your choice of bran (use rice bran if you are gluten-sensitive) and store in an airtight container in the refrigerator.

Breakfast serving suggestion:

> 4 Tablespoons seed mix
> 1 grated apple or pear
> ½ cup yoghurt (cow, goat, sheep or soy)

Blend the seed mix well with yoghurt and then stir in grated fruit.

In winter add the seed mix to cooked oats or rice and eat with warm stewed fruit.

APPENDIX 4

ARTIFICIAL SWEETENERS: ARE THEY SAFE?

Artificial sweeteners found in food products, pharmaceuticals and nutritional supplements include: saccharin, aspartame, sucralose, acesulfame-k, alitame, thaumatin, cyclamates and neotame. Natural sweeteners include: sorbitol, mannitol, stevia (a herb) and fructose.

The research and scientific evaluation behind some of the newer artificial sweeteners is still in very early and inconclusive stages; however, current information on commonly used artificial sweeteners is of great concern.

Saccharine is produced by combining toluene (a distillation of coal tar) with sulphuric acid and ammonia. In other words it is a coal derivative and suspected of giving rise to cancer. It is interesting to note that although saccharine is 300 times sweeter than sugar, neither ants nor houseflies will touch it.

Aspartame, used in the popular artificial sweeteners NutraSweet and Equal, is made up of three components: the amino acids phenylalanine and aspartic acid, and methanol (also known as methyl alcohol or wood alcohol). Methanol is known to be poisonous even when consumed in relatively small amounts. Disorders caused by toxic levels of methanol include blindness, brain swelling and inflammation of the pancreas and heart muscle. In the body methanol metabolises into: formaldehyde, a known carcinogen; formic acid, a carboxylic acid found normally in the venom of bees and ants; and diketopiperazine, which has been shown to cause brain tumours in animals.

A study noted in *Environmental Health Perspectives* (November 2005) reported that rats fed aspartame (at levels that would be the equivalent of the acceptable daily intake for humans) from the age of eight weeks until its natural death showed evidence of malignant cancers including lymphoma, leukemia, and tumours in multiple organs.

Sucralose is produced by chemically changing the structure of the sugar molecule by substituting three chlorine atoms for three hydroxyl groups. In the USA, pre-government approval research showed that sucralose shrunk the thymus gland of rats by up to 40 per cent when taken in large doses. Further studies, however, claim that there is no observable effect on lymphoid organs and the immune system of taking a daily dose of up to 3000 mg of sucralose per kilogram of body weight. Sucralose, under the brand Splenda, has been available on the American market since 1998.

All artificial sweeteners also leave an extremely acidic residue in the body after digestion. Indeed, the acid end-product of their chemical breakdown is more acidic than white sugar.

The message is clear: avoid all sugar substitutes. Either use sugar, at least we know where that comes from – a plant; or better still, avoid all refined sugars and their substitutes completely. We do not need them, it is simply a matter of retraining our taste buds.

APPENDIX : 5

CRISPY TEMPEH WITH AVOCADO AND TAHINI DIP

A delicious way to combine your vegetarian sources of protein and enhance your bowel flora!

1 block tempeh, cut into 15 thin slices
light olive oil for frying
3 tablespoons tahini
juice one small lemon
2 tablespoons chopped fresh coriander
1 avocado
100 gm silken tofu
sea salt

Shallow-fry tempeh slices in olive oil until golden brown and crispy. Drain well. Combine tahini and lemon juice to make a smooth paste and add chopped coriander. Mash avocado and tofu, add a squeeze of lemon and salt to taste. Arrange tempeh on a serving plate and serve with a delicious dollop of each dip.

APPENDIX : 6

HOMEMADE YOGHURT

The following recipe can be used to make cow's-milk, goat's-milk, soy- or rice-milk yoghurt. Be certain to use as your starter a very good-quality yoghurt with an abundance of friendly bacteria, such as *Lactobacillus acidophilus*, *L. bulgaricus* or *L. casei*.

> *500 ml of preferred 'milk' source*
> *2 tablespoons good-quality organic plain yoghurt*

Place the 'milk' in a saucepan and bring to the boil, then let it cool down to approximately 37 °C, or until you can keep your finger in it comfortably for a count of 10. Add the yoghurt, mix thoroughly and pour the mixture into a vacuum flask and seal tightly.

Alternatively, place the mixture into a bowl and cover it with a plate or plastic film; wrap snuggly in a towel or blanket and leave in a warm place, free of draughts. Either method, your yoghurt will be ready in 6–12 hours. Place in the fridge where it will keep for up to a week.

Be sure to save 2 tablespoons from this mixture as a starter for your next yoghurt batch.

APPENDIX 7

....

PROBIOTIC SUPPLEMENTS AND ANTIBIOTICS

Research shows that the probiotic strains of *Lactobacillus rhamnosus*, *L. acidophilus*, *L. casei*, *Bifidobacterium longum* and *B. bifidum* are resistant to 13 commonly prescribed antibiotics:

- Cephalothin
- Gentamicin
- Kanamycin
- Linomycin
- Neomycin
- Nitrofurantoin
- Novobiocin
- Polymyxin B
- Rifampin
- Streptomycin
- Sulfisoxazole
- Tetracycline
- Vancomycin

The message from this research is to take a multi-strain probiotic supplement at the *same* time as antibiotic medication.

APPENDIX 8

....

FIBRE FIGURES

Dietary fibre is the part of plant food that is undigested in the small intestine. There are two types of fibre, soluble and insoluble. Insoluble fibre speeds GIT transit time and promotes regular bowel health. Best sources are: wheat and rice bran, legumes, nuts, seeds and skins of fruit and vegetables. Soluble fibre (it forms a gel when mixed with liquid) lowers serum cholesterol. Best sources are: fruits and vegetables, oat and barley bran, dried beans and peas, flaxseeds and psyllium husks.

Dietary fibre is not substantially broken down by digestive enzymes. Once it reaches the large intestine it undergoes a bacterial fermentation process, which produces short-chain fatty acids (SCFAs). These SCFAs nourish bowel cells, influence the way in which the body uses cholesterol and affect the utilisation of blood sugars. The fibre in food slows down the release of nutrients into the bloodstream, it also contributes to satiety because the fibre bulk fills the stomach and takes longer to eat due to the amount of chewing required.

A dramatic increase in dietary fibre may initially cause some flatulence and discomfort due to the gut fermentation of plant fibres and bran; however, this should not occur if the amount is increased gradually. Aim to eat 30–50 g fibre daily.

FOODS THAT PROVIDE APPROXIMATELY 10 g FIBRE

Only foods of plant origin contain fibre – there is no fibre found in animal proteins, dairy products or eggs.

GRAINS AND CEREALS

2 cups cooked rolled oats

¾ cup whole cooked barley

5–6 biscuits wheat biscuits (e.g. Weet-bix)

½ bran cereal processed

5–6 cups puffed wheat

3 slices rye bread

3 slices high-fibre bran bread

5 slices wholemeal bread

⅔ cup oat bran

1 cup barley bran

½ cup natural bran

3½ cups cooked brown rice

8 cups cooked white rice (easy to see why too much white rice can constipate)

5 cups white pasta (e.g. macaroni)

LEGUMES

1 cup cooked mixed beans

1 cup cooked peas

1 cup baked beans

900 g tofu

1 cup cooked lentils

1 cup cooked chickpeas

NUTS AND SEEDS

100 g almonds

1 cup peanuts

100 g pistachio nuts

¾ cup pecans

¾ cup sunflower seeds

VEGETABLES

3 cups steamed mixed vegetables

2 cups cooked carrots

2 cups cooked cabbage

3 cups cooked broccoli

1 cup steamed spinach

2 cups cooked sweet potato

2–3 medium steamed potatoes with the skin

1 cup broad beans

2 large corn on the cob

FRUIT

3½ medium apples

3 oranges

100 g dried figs

10 dried apricots

3½ bananas

2 passionfruit

400 g blueberries

4 kiwifruit

6 nectarines

2½ pears

6 prunes

200 g raspberries

APPENDIX 9

....

MEADOWSWEET: A FRIEND OF THE DIGESTIVE SYSTEM

Meadowsweet (*Filipendula ulmaria*) is one of my favourite herbs, a kind and generous friend of the digestive system and quite beautiful as well. If you have meadowsweet growing in your herbal patch (and I strongly recommend anyone with tummy troubles should grow this herb in abundance), the best time to pick the fully opened flowers and leaves is mid-to-late summer. Dry gently at a temperature not exceeding 40 °C.

Meadowsweet is a very capable remedy for reducing acidity and inflammation, easing nausea and soothing the mucous membranes of the whole digestive tract. It is especially useful in treating heartburn, gastritis, peptic ulceration, and reduces fever and the pain of inflammatory joint disease.

A tonic I frequently put together in the clinic for clients with abdominal pain, gastric reflux and a touch of nausea is:

30 ml meadowsweet
20 ml cramp bark
25 ml lime blossom (especially good for nervous tension)
25 ml chamomile

Take 5 ml three times a day with meals.

APPENDIX : 10

....

STANDARD ELIMINATION DIET

Daily sample-menu plan
(Choose from Option 1 or Option 2)

Exclude dairy products, wheat, corn, baker's and brewer's yeast,
egg, peanuts, soy, chocolate, orange, tomato and refined sugar.

Pre-breakfast
Glass warm water with lemon juice

Breakfast

Option 1	Option 2
Oat and banana porridge with oat milk or rice milk	2 slices rye sourdough toast topped with ripe mashed banana and dates

Herbal tea

Mid-morning

Piece of fruit in season

Lunch

Option 1	Option 2
100% rye sourdough salad sandwich, add tahini or hummus for extra flavour	Large fresh vegetable salad with handful raw cashews or almonds; or small piece grilled chicken, olive oil/lemon dressing

Herbal tea

Afternoon snack

Option 1	Option 2
Small handful almonds, cashews or sunflower seeds	4–5 dried figs or sun-dried apricots (sulphur-free)

Dinner

Option 1	Option 2
Grilled chicken or fish (use olive oil, and herbs for marinade if desired), julienne of steamed vegetables (include broccoli, carrots, beans, asparagus, zucchini) Dessert: lightly stewed fruit (in own juices) or baked apple stuffed with prunes, dates or figs	Brown rice and lentils or chickpeas, baked vegies of choice (e.g. sweet potato, parsnip, celeriac, carrots, squash) with 1 tsp. cold-pressed flaxseed oil Dessert: fresh fruit in season, e.g. bowl of mixed berries; custard apple and passionfruit

Water as required throughout the day. At least 8 glasses!

APPENDIX : 11

....

GLUTEN-FREE ELIMINATION DIET

Daily sample-menu plan

(Choose from Option 1 or Option 2)

Exclude all the gluten-containing grains: wheat plus rye, barley and oats,
plus those foods excluded in the Standard Elimination Diet.

Pre-breakfast
Glass warm water with lemon juice

Breakfast

Option 1	Option 2
Buckwheat and banana porridge with rice milk *or* Buckwheat pancakes topped with banana	3–4 tbsp. seed mix (use rice bran as bran component), grated apple, moisten with apple/pear juice

Weak lemon tea or other herbal tea of choice

Mid-morning

Glass carrot, beetroot and cucumber juice; if too difficult plain carrot juice is fine

Lunch

Option 1	Option 2
Lentil or vegie burger and salad *or* Homemade vegetable soup with rice or millet	Baked potato in jacket with tahini or hummus topping, large salad – include plenty of rocket, endive, cucumber and beetroot plus small handful raw cashews or almonds, flaxseed oil/lemon juice dressing

Herbal tea (as per breakfast)

Afternoon snack

Fresh berries (in season) or pear

Dinner

Option 1	Option 2
Kidney or adzuki beans with brown rice, steamed vegies with 2 tsp. cold-pressed flaxseed oil, tahini/lemon dressing Dessert: baked apple stuffed with prunes	Grilled chicken or fish seasoned with fennel and lemon, stir-fried asparagus, zucchini, green beans and broccoli in cold-pressed olive oil Dessert: fresh fruit in season, e.g. cherries, apricots, peaches

Water as required throughout the day. At least 8 glasses!

APPENDIX : 12

....

FOOD CHALLENGE DIARY

	FOOD CHALLENGED (1 type of food only)	SYMPTOMS (e.g. moodiness, abdominal pain, irritable bowel, itchy skin, runny nose,
BREAKFAST (single serving challenge food)		
LUNCH (1–2 servings challenge food)		
DINNER (2–3 servings challenge food)		

PULSE RATE BEFORE & AFTER CHALLENGE
(beats per min)

Before challenge .... bpm

5 minutes after .... bpm

10 minutes after .... bpm

Before challenge .... bpm

5 minutes after .... bpm

10 minutes after .... bpm

Before challenge .... bpm

5 minutes after .... bpm

10 minutes after .... bpm

APPENDIX : 13

WHEAT SOURCES

Those of you who have attempted a wheat-exclusion diet on the road to good health would have discovered how insidious this grain is. It is often found lurking in 'benign' stock cubes and even soy milk (think malt), and can even be discovered sneakily lolling around in rye sour-dough and children's sweets! Outrageous, indeed. To help you avoid this problematic grain, I have put together a comprehensive but by no means exhaustive list of possible wheat sources. No excuses now for any slip-ups on your wheat-exclusion diet!

Flour, bread, pasta, cereals, noodles, biscuits, cakes, breadcrumbs, spelt, kamut, couscous, burghul, semolina, tritacale, wheatgerm, wheat bran, soy sauce, thickener added to soups and salad dressings, malt, soups with noodles or spaghetti, imitation meat products (such as gluten dishes found in some Asian cuisines), hot dogs, imitation crab meat, ice-cream, ice-cream cones, cottage cheese with modified starch, licorice, beverages such as beer, ale, malted milks, cereal coffee substitute, Worcestershire sauce, MSG, modified food starch, vegetable starch, natural flavouring.

The lesson is clear: always read the food label. The less processed the food the better as there is less opportunity for unwanted and unnecessary wheat additives.

Note: of the 8000 species in the grass family, only a small number play a significant role in the human diet. Other than sugar cane, the cereals are: wheat, barley, rye and oats.

APPENDIX : 14

....

A GUIDE TO GLUTEN

Gluten is the main protein component of the cereal grains: wheat, durum wheat, rye, barley, oats and triticale. Semolina, bulgur, kamut, couscous and spelt, being wheat derivatives or relatives, also contain gluten.

Many foods include these grains, such as pasta, noodles, breakfast cereals, breads, biscuits and cakes. It is also found hidden in malt extract and flavourings, thickeners, breadcrumbs and other additives. Examples of foods that may contain *hidden* gluten are sausages, curry powders, batters, yeast extract, soy sauces, malt vinegars, soy milks, beer, licorice, baking powder, icing sugars – it's everywhere! Check all ingredients on the food label if in doubt.

Gluten-free grains are: *rice, corn, millet, buckwheat, amaranth, quinoa, sorghum and teff.*

Flour made from the following foods are also gluten-free: *soy, lupin, lentil, potato and pea.*

Ingredients that are wheat derived, but *do not* contain gluten are: glucose, dextrose, caramel colour (150), sorbitol and maltitol (965).

Note: be careful to check for gluten in seemingly benign products such as envelopes, stamps, crayons, playdough and medicines.

APPENDIX : 15

PROTEIN COMBINATIONS FOR VEGETARIANS

Protein sources for vegetarians include: grains, legumes, seeds and nuts, and vegetables. These sources are considered 'incomplete' proteins because each food group misses one or two of the essential amino acids. Legumes, for example, are low in methionine, and grains are low in lysine. Therefore it is necessary to combine our vegetarian protein sources wisely to obtain a complete vegetarian protein component. Recommended combinations:

- grains and legumes, e.g. rice and lentils or beans and taco shells
- seeds or nuts and legumes, e.g. tempeh and tahini or hummus (i.e. chickpeas and sesame seeds)
- grains and nuts or seeds, e.g. linseed and sunflower toast with almond spread.

APPROXIMATE LEVELS OF PROTEIN IN POPULAR FOODS:

meat (100 g)	20–25 g	milk/yoghurt (1 cup)	8 g
fish (100 g)	15–20 g	egg (1)	6 g
beans/legumes (1 cup)	7.5–15 g	cheese (30 g)	6–8 g
whole grains (1 cup)	5–12 g	vegetables/fruits (1 cup)	2–4 g

The recommended daily allowance of protein is 0.8 g per kilo of 'ideal' body weight; for example, a female weighing 50 kg requires 40 g of protein a day, and a male weighing 70 kg requires 56 g a day.

Note: a simple way to increase the amount of protein in your meals is to add a handful of red or green lentils to the pot whenever you cook brown rice or barley.

APPENDIX | 16

....

HOW TO MAKE THAT (HERBAL) MEDICINE GO DOWN!

Being a naturopath and herbalist can make one a little immune to the taste of some herbs, but I have to agree that a few herbs, particularly those astringent herbs used in formulas to treat ulcers, can be a little on the nose . . . and tongue. So, here are a few tips for getting those very therapeutic herbs down painlessly and quickly. Swigging it neat followed by a glass of water is the easiest method, but I can already hear the cries of 'but it's awful!', so if in pain try the following:

- Dilute the 5 ml dose with about 10 ml water or fruit juice. Swallow quickly in one go as this reduces contact time with taste buds.
- For very sensitive individuals, try sucking on some ice beforehand to deaden the taste buds and the olfactory nerve, or chill the entire bottle of herbal medicine by storing in the fridge.
- After swallowing the medicine, immediately rinse your mouth with water. The best method is to hold the diluted herbs in one hand, and the water to rinse with in the other. The two liquids are then consumed in a one-two action, as quickly as possible (thanks to Kerry Bone for the one-two method).

However, most clients actually *grow to love their herbs* and, by the time we are ready to discontinue, are sad to see them go (it's true!).

REFERENCES

Allergy Advisor <http://www.allergyadvisor.com/Educational>.

Atkinson, R., *Modern Naturopathy and Age-old Healers*, Harper & Row, Sydney, 1986, p. 76.

Atkinson, W., Sheldon, T.A., et Al., 'Food Elimination Based on IgG Antibodies in IBS', *Gut*, vol. 53, no. 10, October 2004, pp. 1459–64.

Ash, Michael, 'All Diseases Begin in the Gut', BioCeutical (Teleconference) Seminar, October 2005.

Balch, J.F., *The Super Anti-oxidants*, M. Evans & Co., New York, 1998, p. 213.

Balch, P.A., *Prescription for Nutritional Healing*, Avery Publishing, New York, 1997, pp. 47, 217, 223, 423.

Bettelheim, F., Brown, W.H. & March, J., *Introduction to General, Organic and Biochemistry*, Brooks/Cole, New York, 1995, p. 618.

BioCeuticals Clinical Insights, 'Allergies', vol. 4, March 2005, p. 1.

BioCeuticals Clinical Insights, 'Allergies 2', vol. 5, April 2005, p. 5.

BioCeuticals Clinical Insights, 'Inflammatory Bowel Disease', vol. 12, November 2005, p. 3.

BioCeuticals Clinical Insights, 'Metabolic Syndrome', vol. 14, January 2006, p. 1.

BioCeuticals Clinical Insights, 'Symbiosis: The Future of Probiotics', vol. 25, May 2002, pp. 1–8.

BioCeuticals Clinical Insights, 'Weight Management', vol. 2, January 2005, pp. 1–4.

BioConcepts, 'Confused about Probiotics', *Bulletin*, Issue 2, 2005, pp. 6–10.

BioConcepts, 'Mood Disorders Therapeutic Guidelines', 2006, pp. 3–12.

BioConcepts Professional Papers, 'Brain Anti-oxidants Protocol'. 2005.

BioConcepts Seminar Notes, 'The Brain-gut Connection', 2005.

Blackmores Seminar Notes, 'Gut Feelings: The Multifunctional Role of the GIT', November 2005.

Bland, Jeffery, 'Neurochemistry: A New Paradigm for Managing Brain Biochemical Disturbances', *Journal of Orthomolecular Medicine*, vol 9, no. 3, 1994.

Brighthope, Dr. Ian, 'Lactose and Lactose Intolerance', *Nutrition Care Bulletin*, April 2006, p. 1.

Byun T., Kofod L., Blinkovsky, A., *Journal of Agricultural and Food Chemistry*, vol. 49, no. 4, pp. 2061–63, April 2001.

Buist, Robert, 'Solving Wheat and Dairy Problems', Seminar Notes, 2003, pp. 2–16.

Burgess, N., 'Holistic Approaches to Treating IBS' (www.dnagroup.net.au).

The Eagle Vision , 'The Vicious Cycle of Insulin Resistance', vol. 23, April/May 2005, pp. 2–12.

Edwards, C. et al., *Davidson's Principles and Practice of*

Medicine, Churchill Livingston, New York, 1995, pp. 456–8.

Everyday Health Magazine, 'Allergies, the Facts', Autumn 2006, p. 41.

Fisher, Leslie, *The Clinical Science of Mineral Therapy*, Maurice Blackmore Research Foundation, Balgowlah, Sydney, 1993, p. 53.

Galland, Leo, 'Leaky Gut Syndromes: Breaking the Vicious Cycle', *HealthWorld Online*, <http://www.healthy.net>.

Gartner, R. et al., 'Selenium Supplementation in Patients with Autoimmune Thyroiditis', *Journal of Clinical Endocrinology and Metabolism*, vol. 87, no. 4, 2002, pp. 1687–91.

Gill, S.R., et al., *Science*, vol. 312, 2006, pp. 1355–1359.

Haas, E., *Staying Healthy with Nutrition*, Celestial Arts Publishing, California, 1992, pp. 128, 257, 397, 873.

Halliday, Jess, 'Broccoli Compounds Slow Bladder Cancer in Lab', 29 July 2005, <http://www.nutraingredients.com>.

Hoffman, D., *The New Holistic Herbal*, Element Books, London, 1992, pp. 53, 215.

Journal of Complementary Medicine, vol. 4, no. 6, November/ December 2005, p. 68.

Journal of Complementary Medicine, vol. 5, no. 1, January/ February 2006, pp. 12–22.

Journal of Complementary Medicine, 'IBS', vol. 5, no. 1, January/February 2006, p. 12.

Journal of Complementary Medicine, vol. 5, no. 3, May/June 2006, p. 72.

Journal of Complementary Medicine, vol. 5, June/July 2006, p. 104.

Journal of Complementary Medicine Journal Digest, March/April 2006, p. 24.

Journal Functional Medicine, 'Intestinal Harmony Through Symbiosis', vol. 23, April 2002, pp. 2-4.

Journal Functional Medicine, 'Controversy surrounds Sweeteners', vol. 29, November 2003, p. 12.

Journal Functional Medicine, 'Prodophilus In-vitro Testing', vol. 32, June/July 2004, p. 16.

Journal Functional Medicine, 'Obesity: A Worldwide Epidemic', vol. 39, October–December 2005, pp. 6–7.

Journal Functional Medicine, vol. 41, March/April 2006, pp. 4–6, 6–12.

Journal of Pediatric Psychology, vol. 25, no. 4, 2000, pp. 225–54.

Journal of Pediatrics, vol. 145, no. 5, November 2004, pp. 606–11.

Konturek, S.J., et al., 'Neuroendocrinology of the Pancreas: Role of Brain-gut Axis in Pancreatic Secretion', *European Journal of Pharmacology*, vol. 481, 2003, pp. 1–14.

Linus Pauling Institute, <http://.lpi.oregonstate.edu>.

McCance, K. & Huetter, E., *Pathophysiology: The Biologic Basis for Disease in Adults and Children*, Mosby, Missouri, 1994, pp. 300–305, 1282–1325.

McCarty, M., 'Magnesium May Mediate the Favorable

Impact of Whole Grains on Insulin Sensitivity', *Medical Hypotheses*, vol. 64, no. 3, 2005, pp. 619–625.

McGee, Harold, *On Food and Cooking*, Scribner, New York, 2004, pp. 14, 461, 521.

McGrath, Melanie L., et al, 'Impirically Supported Treatments in Pediatric Psychology, Constipation and Encopresis', *Journal of Pediatrics*, vol. 25, no. 4, 2000, pp. 225–54.

McMillin, D.L., et al., 'The Abdominal Brain and Enteric Nervous System', *The Journal of Alternative and Complementary Medicine*, vol. 5, no. 6, 1999.

Magee, E.A., Edmond, L.M., et al., 'Associations Between Diet and Disease Activity in Ulcerative Colitis Patients Using a Novel Method of Data Analysis', *Nutrition Journal*, vol. 4, no. 1, 2005, p. 7.

MD Consult <http://www.mdconsult.com>.

Mediherb Professional Review, 'Gymnema sylvestre', no. 75, April 2001.

Metagenics, 'Choosing the Best Supplement for Your Patients', *Update*, October/November 2005, pp. 2–4.

Metagenics, 'Chronic Disease and Mucosal Immunology', *Update*, August/September 2003, part 2, p. 10.

Metagenics, 'Clinical Approaches to Curbing the Cravings', *Update*, January 2006, pp. 10–11.

Metagenics, 'Clinical Digestion and Assimilation of Zinc', *Update*, February/March 2006, p. 6.

Metagenics, *Immunology Key Clinical Concepts*, p. 43.

Metagenics, 'Pre and Probiotic', *Research Literature Review*, 2004.

Metagenics, 'Treat Strains Differently', *Update*, April/May 2006, pp. 6–7.

Metagenics Seminar Notes, 'How to Keep the Fat Off', February 2005, p. 6.

Mills, S., *The Essential Book of Herbal Medicine*, Penguin, London, 1991.

Mills, S. & Bone, K., *The Essential Guide to Herbal Medicine*, Churchill Livingston, Missouri, 2005, p. 437.

Murray, M., *The Complete Book of Juicing*, Prima Publishing, California, 1992, p. 39.

Myers, S. & Hawrelak, J., 'The Causes of Intestinal Dysbiosis: A Review', *Alternative Medicine Review*, June 2004.

New Developments in Functional Toxicology and Gastrointestinal Rehabilitation, seminar notes, May 2002.

Nutrition Care Bulletin, 'Antibacterial Activity of Hydrolyzable Tannins', vol. 13, issue 6, December 2005/ January 2006, p. 3.

Nutrition Care Bulletin, 'The Gluten Gut', David Kirk ed., vol. 13, issue 3, June/July 2005, pp. 1–3.

Nutrition Care Bulletin, 'Integral Nutrition', vol. 13, issue 1, February 2005, pp. 1–4.

Rachman, Dr Brad, 'Unique Features of Non-animal Derived Enzymes', seminar notes.

Robinson, R., 'Physiological Effects of Arabinogalactans in

Healthy Men and Women', graduate thesis, University of
Minnesota, 1999.

Sach, J.A. & Chang, L., 'IBS Current Treatment Options',
Gastroenterology, vol. 5, no. 4, August 2002,
pp. 267–278.

Sakamoto, N., S. Kono, et al., 'Dietary Risk Factors for
Inflammatory Bowel Disease: a Multi-centre Case-control
Study in Japan', *Journal of Inflammatory Bowel Disease*,
vol. 11, no. 2, 2005, pp. 154–159.

Seyle, Hans, *Stress in Health and Disease*, Butterworths,
London, 1976.

Smith, Jennifer & Coulson, Samantha, 'Pathology Testing for
Mood Disorders', *Orthoplex Bulletin*, vol. 2, 2005.

Stuttaford, Dr Thomas, 'Gut Feelings Signals a Worry',
Weekend Australian, Weekend Health section,
10–11 December 2005, p. 21.

Weekend Australian, Weekend Health section, 'The Pulse',
23 Jan 2005, p. 22.

Weekend Australian, Weekend Health section, 'The Pulse',
22–23 April 2006, p. 21.

Weekend Australian, Weekend Health section, 'The Pulse',
3–4 June 2006, p. 21.

Weiss, Rudolf, *Herbal Medicine*, Beaconsfield Publishers,
Stuttgart, 1994, p. 58.

Index

abdominal breathing 27
abdominal massage 76, 78
abdominal pain 4, 26, 208–9
absorption of nutrients 14
acetylcholine 20
acne 99
adaptogenic herbs 27
adrenal glands 23, 26, 169
adrenalin 106, 109, 170
adverse food reactions 102–15
aerobic bacteria 56
aflatoxin 64
agrimony 34
alcohol 5, 33, 35, 38, 56, 57
alimentary canal see GIT
allergies (sensitivities)
  anaphylactic shock 103
  definition 102–3
  'delayed' hypersensitivity 103
  detection 103, 106, 107–11
  effects on gut 5, 33, 46
  and food cravings 106, 107
  hypersensitivity 102–3
  and peptic ulcers 188, 191
  signs and symptoms 104–6
  spaced out feeling 143
allergies see food allergies
aloe vera 34, 79, 189–90, 206
aluminium 152, 153
Alzheimer's disease 153
amines 16
amino acids 25–6
amylase 9, 122
anaemia 123
anaerobic bacteria 56–7
anal sphincter 15, 71
anaphylactic shock 103
Andre, Claude 130
androgens 16
antacids 152–3, 187
anthraquinone glucosides 79

antibiotics
  causing diarrhoea 33, 94–5
  and gut flora 56, 57, 59, 67–8
  link with IBS 25
  probiotics with 67–8, 220
  thrush following 95
anticholinergics 36
anti-depressants 20, 36
anti-nutrients 61–2
anti-oxidants 64, 131, 160, 190
anus 10, 14–15
appendicitis 73
appendix 10, 14
arabinogalactans 57–8
arthritis 130
artificial sweeteners 33, 216–17
ascending colon 10, 14
aspartame 216–17
assessory organs 7, 17–18
atopic dermatitis 62

Bach flowers 98
Bach Rescue Remedy 26–7, 98
bacteria
  aerobic bacteria 56
  anaerobic bacteria 56–7
  causing ulcers 187–8
  gas-producing 45
  see also gut flora
bad breath 74, 132–9
bananas 192
basal body temperature 157
basal metabolic rate (BMR) 156
bayberry 34, 93
Bifidobacterium 27, 65
  action 62–3
  antibiotic-resistant 67–8
  B. adolentis 64
  B. bifidum 63, 64, 220
  B. breve 63, 64
  B. lactis 77, 132, 207
  B. longum 63, 64, 66, 67, 220

  in large intestine 15, 56–7, 62
  making your own 63–4
  and stress 24
bile 3, 14, 17
bioflavonoids 190
biotin 63
bitter foods 147
bladderwrack 167–8
bloating 1–2
  alleviating 62–3, 208–9
  case study 48–53
  causes 12, 24, 46–8, 54, 74
  gas production 45–6
  trigger foods 47
blood sugar levels 18
blood test for sensitivities 107–9
BMR (basal metabolic rate) 156
body temperature 157
bolus 11
bowel motions 15
  daily 69–70
  good bowel habits 72–3, 210–11
  mechanics of 71–2
  normal 70
  regular 70, 87
  transit time test 70–1
brain-gut connection 19–28
bread, toasting 50
breakfast 82–3, 199–200
breast milk 62
bromelain 26, 146, 151

cabbage juice 131, 189
caffeine 33, 35, 83–4
calcium 26, 93, 122, 123–4
calendula 195
cAMP see cyclic adenosine monophosphate
Candida albicans 61, 64, 65
carbohydrates
  digestible 14
  fermentation 16
  non-digestible 57–8
carbohydrate intolerance 143

carbonated drinks 35, 42, 47
carrageenan 179
cecum 10, 14, 91
cereals 222
CFS see chronic fatigue syndrome
challenge diary 110, 111
chamomile 27, 34, 35, 92, 93, 192, 208
charcoal tablets 47–8, 75
chewing food 8–9, 35, 76, 122, 147
chewing gum 35, 45
chlorophyll 138
cholesterol 17
chromium 26, 161, 163–4, 165
chronic fatigue syndrome (CFS) 103, 130
chyme 14
Clostridium perfringens 61
Cnidium 167
coeliac disease 5, 130
  diagnosis 116–17, 118–19
  genetic predisposition 116, 117
  signs and symptoms 116, 118–19
  silent presenters 118
  treatment 120–4
coenzyme Q10 134–5
coffee 5, 33
cola nut allergen 52
Coleus 166–7
colon 10, 15, 24–5
colonic irrigation 80–1
complete digestive stool analysis (CDSA) 214
constipation 70
  case study 81–8
  causes 41, 75–6
  chronic 15, 74
  good bowel habits 72–3, 210–11
  and halitosis 74, 132, 135–9
  rebound 48, 75
  skin problems 85
  spastic 41
  symptoms 73–4
  treatment 34–5, 75–81
copper 17
cortisol 88, 106, 169

cow's milk 191
  allergy to 113
  see also lactose intolerance
creatine 170
Crohn's disease (regional enteritis) 177
  case study 181–5
  and depression 25
  effects on gut 5, 178
  foods implicated in 179
  and leaky gut syndrome 130
  symptoms 178–9
  treatment 61, 62, 131, 181
cyclic adenosine monophosphate (cAMP) 166–7

dairy foods 47
dandelion root 35, 77, 207
deep-diaphragmatic breathing 76
defecation 15, 62
defecation reflex 71
'delayed' hypersensitivity 103
Dermatitis herpetiformis 118
descending colon 10, 14
diabetes 134, 169
diarrhoea
  antibiotic-associated 33, 94–5
  case study 98–101
  causes 90–1
  diet-related 92
  parasitic 95–6
  rebound 94–5
  stress-associated 97–8
  treatment 34–5, 91–8
  what is it? 89–90
digestive enzymes 8, 13, 65, 140–1, 143, 213, 221
  encouraging production 144–7
  enzyme supplements 149–50
  law of adaptive secretion of enzymes 145, 151
digestive system 19, 207
  components 8–18
  function 7

diverticulitis 73
duodenal ulcer 151, 186, 187–8
duodenum 10, 11, 13, 17
dysbiosis 143

eating quickly 33
Eaton, Keith 144
echinacea 195
EFA see essential fatty acids
elimination diet
  gluten-free 121–2, 225
  standard 224
ELISA see enzyme linked immuno-sorbent assay test
endorphins 21, 28, 106
enkephalins 20–1, 28
enteric nervous system 19–20
enzymes
  getting the most from 150–1
  insufficiency 140–1
  law of adaptive secretion of enzymes 145, 151
  metabolic 141
  plant 149–50
  proteolytic 150
  in raw foods 145
  supplements 122, 149–50
  see also digestive enzymes
enzyme linked immuno-sorbent assay test (ELISA) 109
epsom salts 79
Escherichia coli 56, 58, 61
essential fatty acids (EFA) 122–3, 171, 191
exercise 28, 72, 76, 87, 154, 171, 211
exorphins 142–3

faecal mass 15, 16
fats 14, 17, 155
fermentation 12, 16, 45
fibre 4
  and bloating 47
  and bowel habit 72
  fermentation 16
  foods for 221–2

insoluble 221
soluble 35, 221
fizzy drinks 33
flare-and-wheal reaction
103
flatulence 45, 63
flaxseed meal 34
folate 26
folic acid 63, 64, 183,
206
food allergies *see* allergies
(sensitivities)
food challenge diary
226–7
food elimination and
challenge test 110–11
food intolerance 24,
104–5
forskolin 166–7
FOS *see* fructo-
oligosaccharides
free radicals 129, 131, 160
fringe tree cramp bark
35, 77, 93, 207–8
fructo-oligosaccharides
(FOS) 57, 58
fructose (levulose) 14, 35,
37, 113–14
and bloating 46
malabsorption 113,
114, 115
fructose-malabsorption
test 37
fruit
containing fibre 222
on empty stomach 146

Galen 3
gallbladder 7, 10, 14, 17
gas production 45–6
gastric juice 8, 9, 12–13
gastric mucosa 23
gastric ulcer 131, 151, 186,
187–8
gastrointestinal tract
(GIT) 3, 61
allergic reactions in
104
assessory organs 7,
17–18
components 7, 8–17
crimes against 4–5
gas production 45–6
permeability 128
and stress 20–1, 22–5
transit time 70

see also gut flora; gut-
brain connection;
leaky gut syndrome;
peristalsis
general adaptation
syndrome 23
ginger 35
GIT *see* gastrointestinal
tract
globe artichoke 35, 77,
210
glucose
and insulin 18
metabolism 14, 18,
163–4, 170
glucose intolerance 164
glucose tolerance factors
(GTF) 163, 164
glutamic acid 164
glutamine 127, 130, 131,
188, 190, 206
glutathione 131
gluten 111, 119, 124–5, 229
gluten sensitivity *see*
coeliac disease
gluten-free diet 121–2, 225
glycine 164
goitrogenic foods 166,
175
golden seal 194
golden staph
(*Staphylococcus
aureus*) 61, 62
gota kola 27, 171, 193, 205
grains 222
GTF *see* glucose tolerance
factors
gum disease 134–5
gut *see* gastrointestinal
tract (GIT)
gut flora 14, 25, 46
and antibiotics 56,
57, 59
imbalance 16, 54, 143
implanted at birth
55–6
numbers 55
pain-free gut protocol
205–11
role 15–16, 56
treating imbalance 27,
57–65
gut–brain connection
19–28, 137
gymnema 164

haemorrhoids 74
hair loss 171–2
halitosis 74
case study 135–9
causes 132–3
foods contributing to
132–3
gum disease 134–5
morning breath 133–4
and saliva production
132, 133–4
tongue scraping 133, 134
hard palate 8
HCl *see* hydrochloric acid
Healthy Gut Guide diet
breakfast 199–200
daily dietary essentials
198–9
dessert 202
dinner 201–2
herbal teas 203
lunch 200–1
portion sizes 203–5
snacks 202–3
supplements 206–7
tips 205
water 203
Helicobacter pylori 187–
8, 189, 190, 191–2
herbal medicine
adaptogenic herbs 27
anti-parasitic 96–7
laxatives 79–80
nervine herbs 193
supporting thyroid
166–8
taking 231
teas 208–10
see also particular
conditions
Hippocrates 2–3
histamine 20
hormones
gastric 12
thyroid-releasing
(TRH) 156–7, 161,
167
Howell, Dr Edward 141
hydrochloric acid (HCl)
3, 5
in gastric secretion 12,
13, 14
testing for deficiency
147
and ulcer medications
13

hydrogen breath test 114
hypochlorhydria 140–1
  and bacterial
    overgrowth 143
  causes 144
  mineral therapy for
    151–2
  signs and symptoms
    141–2
  treatment 151–2
hypotension 174
hypothyroidism 156–9

IBD *see* inflammatory
  bowel disease
IBS *see* irritable bowel
  syndrome
ileocecal valve 15
ileum 10, 13
immune system 3, 56, 61,
  128–9
inflammatory bowel
  disease (IBD)
  case study 181–5
  causes 177–8
  and diet 178
  drug therapy 178
  and smoking 178
  treatment 61, 62, 181
  see also Crohn's
    disease; ulcerative
    colitis
insulin 18, 170
intestinal flora *see* gut
  flora
intestinal massage 76, 78
intestinal parasites 5, 95–6
intrinsic factor 12
inulin 58
iodine 155, 158–9
iron 17, 122, 123, 190
irritable bowel syndrome
  (IBS)
  and antibiotics 25
  case studies 36–43
  causes 23, 25, 32–3
  changes in gut flora 24
  and depression 25
  diagnosis 31–2
  meaning 29–30
  signs and symptoms 31
  treatment 32, 34–6, 62
isothiocyanates 166

jejunum 10, 13

lactase 61, 112–13
lactase deficiency 59
Lactobacillus 55, 56, 64
  action 61–2
  antibiotic-resistant
    67–8
  L. acidophilus 35, 56,
    60, 61, 66, 67, 92,
    207, 220
  L. bulgaricus 60
  L. casei 59, 60, 62,
    66, 220
  L. plantarum 35, 36,
    59, 61–2, 66
  L. rhamnosus 62, 66,
    67, 95, 220
  L. salivarius 62
  and stress 24
lactose intolerance 46,
  61, 100, 104, 111–13
large intestine 7, 13
  bacteria in 15–16, 56
  components 7
  fermentation in 12, 16
  waste storage 73
  water absorption in 16
law of adaptive secretion
  of enzymes 145, 151
laxatives 36, 78–80
leaky gut syndrome 5
  associated conditions
    24, 129–30
  stress as a cause 23–4,
    128
  symptoms 129–30
  testing for 130
  treatment 130–1
legumes 46, 222
lemon balm 34, 77
leptin 169
levulose *see* fructose
licorice root 188–9
lifestyle and constipation
  75–7
lime flowers 27, 77, 207
lingual lipase 9
lipids 16
lipogenesis 155
liver 7, 10
  bile production 14, 17
  detoxifier 17, 128–9
  free radical production
    129
  herbal teas for 207
  and immune system
    128–9

metabolism in 14
  protein breakdown 17
  vitamin storage 17
lymphatic system 23, 87

McGee, Harold 112
magnesium 26, 35, 51, 77,
  88, 93, 122, 126, 169,
  170–1, 206
magnesium aspartate 171
magnesium orotate 171
marshmallow 93, 193–4
masseter muscles 8–9
meadowsweet 34, 92, 93,
  193, 208, 223
measuring portions
  204–5
meat 12, 46
metabolic enzymes 141
metabolic rate 154–6,
  168–71
metabolic syndrome 163
metabolism, sluggish
  154–5
  case study 171–6
  treatment for 158–69
migraine 73
milk of magnesia 79
morning breath 133–4
mouth 7, 8–9

nails 38, 100, 172
naturally fermented
  foods 59
nervine herbs 193
nervous system 3, 137
  enteric 19–20
  peripheral 19–20
neurotransmitters 20,
  24–6
non-coeliac gluten
  intolerance (sub-
  clinical gluten
  sensitivity) 124–6
non-steroidal anti-
  inflammatory drugs
  (NSAIDs) 187
noradrenalin 20
norepinephrine 159
NSAIDs *see* non-
  steroidal anti-
  inflammatory drugs
nuts and seeds 222

oats 119–20
oesophagus 7, 10, 11

oestrogen 16
oligosaccharides 63
Omega 3 and 6 essential
fatty acids 122–3
oral contraceptive 56, 57
osteomalacia 153
osteoporosis 123–4
osthol 167
overeating 154
oxygen 45

pain medications 33
pain-free gut protocol
205–11
palm method of
measuring portions
204–5
pancreas 7, 10, 17–18
pancreatic enzymes 3,
207
pancreatic insufficiency
5, 140
causes 144
signs of 142
treatment 144–53
papain 146, 151
parasitic diarrhoea 95–6
Parkinson's disease 153
parotid glands 9
pelvic floor muscles 15
peppermint 34, 35
pepsin 13, 14
pepsinogen 12, 13
peptic ulcer 5, 23, 186–8,
191
see also duodenal
ulcer; gastric ulcer
peptides 106
peripheral nervous system
19–20
peristalsis 8, 11, 15, 21,
71, 72
manual stimulation 78
pharynx 7, 11
phenylalaline 25–6
phytates 162
Pilates 27, 76
pineapple sensitivity 146
pituitary-thyroid axis 167
plant enzyme
supplements 149–50
potassium 93, 122
potassium chloride 12,
151–2
prebiotics
arabinogalactans 57–8

fructo-oligosaccharides
57, 58
probiotics 27, 36, 63, 77,
97, 191–2
additives 67
with antibiotics 67–8,
220
arabinogalactans 57–8
binders 67
effective dose 66
food sources 58–60
fructo-oligosaccharides
57, 58
human origin 66–7
maximising effect
65–8
storing 68
strains 60–5
see also
Bifidobacterium;
Lactobacillus;
particular
conditions
*Propionibacterium
freudenreichii* 64
protein 16, 17
becomes amino acids
13, 14
not mixing with fruit
12
in popular foods 230
vegetarian protein
combinations 230
Prout, William 13
psyllium 47, 58, 92–3
pulse test 109
pyloric sphincter 11

RAST (blood test) 103,
107
raw foods 145, 189
rebound constipation
48, 75
rebound diarrhoea 94–5
recipes
anti-ulcer herbal tonic
195–6
crispy tempeh with
avocado and tahini
dip 218
dukkahish dip 165–6
enzyme-enhancing
salad 148–9
homemade yoghurt 219
rehydration soup 93–4
seed mix 215

for sluggish digestion
and liver 210
rectal reflex 71
rectum 8, 10, 14–15, 71
regional enteritis *see*
Crohn's disease
rehydration 93–4
rheumatoid arthritis 128

saccharine 216
Saccharomyces boulardii
64–5, 95
St Mary's thistle 77, 207
saliva 98
and halitosis 132,
133–4
role 8, 9
salivary glands 7, 9
Salmonella typhimurium
61
salt tablets 93
satiety 12, 154–5, 169
sauerkraut 59
SCFA *see* short-chain
fatty acids
seaweed 158–9
seeds and nuts 222
selenium 160–1, 165
self-prescribing 26
Selye, Hans 23
senna 78–9
sensitivities *see* allergies
serotonin 20–2, 26, 112,
137, 155
short-chain fatty acids
(SCFA) 16, 56, 57, 221
Siberian ginseng 27, 171,
193, 205
sigmoid colon 10, 14, 15
skin 85, 130
skin-prick test 103, 107
skullcap 27
slippery elm 34, 93, 94,
100, 130, 153, 189, 196
small intestine 7, 11, 56
components 10, 13
and digestion 13
regeneration of lining
14
villi 13
smoking 33, 38, 187
sodium 93
sodium phosphate 151–2
soft palate 8
sourdough bread 59
soy 59

soy milk 101
spastic constipation 41
sphincters 11, 15, 71
spicy foods 5, 33
sports drinks 99
sprue *see* coeliac disease
Staphylococcus aureus
    (golden staph) 61, 62
starches 9, 16
starvation and metabolic
    rate 168–9
steatorrhoea 118
steroids 187
stomach 7, 10
    gastric juice 8, 9, 12–13
    mucosa 23
    ulcers 131, 151, 186,
        187–8
stools
    analysis 96, 214
    in diarrhoea 89–90
    'softeners' 36, 78–80
*Streptococcus
    thermophilus* 64, 67
stress
    effects on gut 4, 5, 13,
        22–5, 33, 41, 56–7,
        97–8, 128, 187
    and enzyme
        production 144
    and exercise 171
    and metabolic rate
        169–71
    and weight gain
        169–70
stress management 26–7,
    35, 170–1, 193, 205–6
stressors 23
sub-clinical gluten
    sensitivity (non-coeliac
    gluten intolerance)
    124–6
sub-clinical
    hypothyroidism 157
substance P 20, 24, 26
sucralose 217
sugar 56
sulphur-containing foods
    35, 45–6
supplements 206–7
    enzymes 149–50
    see also particular
        conditions;
        particular minerals;
        prebiotics;
        probiotics; vitamins

swimming 76
Syndrome X 163

T3 (triiodothyronine) 155
T4 (thyroxine) 155
tannin 34
taste buds 9
tea 5, 33, 84
teeth 7
tempeh 59
thermogenesis 154, 155–6
thrush 61, 64, 65, 81, 95
thymus 23
thyroid gland
    and body temperature
        157
    goitrogenic foods 166,
        175
    hormone production
        155–6
    hypothyroidism 156–9
    and metabolic rate 154
    and thermogenesis
        155–6
thyroid-releasing
    hormone (TRH) 156–
    7, 161, 167
thyroxine (T4) 155
toilet, how to sit on
    72–3, 76
tongue 7, 8, 99
    scraping 133, 134
    taste buds 9
transverse colon 10, 14
TRH *see* thyroid-
    releasing hormone
triglycerides 9
triiodothyronine (T3) 155
tryptophan 25–6
tyrosine 25–6, 155, 158,
    159–60

ulcerative colitis 5, 177
    diagnosing 180
    dietary factors in
        180–1
    and leaky gut
        syndrome 130
    symptoms 180
    treatment 61, 131, 181
ulcers *see* duodenal ulcer;
    gastric ulcer; peptic
    ulcer

vegetables
    fibre in 222

gas-producing 45–6
organic 148
overcooking 50
raw 145, 189
vegetarian protein
    combinations 230
vegetarians 173
verbena 77
vervain 27, 207
villi 13
vitamin A 17
vitamin B group 26, 56,
    63, 77, 91, 97, 101, 122,
    126, 206
vitamin B1 26
vitamin B2 26
vitamin B3 26, 164
vitamin B5 26, 170–1
vitamin B6 26, 170–1
vitamin B12 12–13, 17, 64,
    123, 206
vitamin C 26, 125, 170–1,
    188
vitamin D 17
vitamin E 17, 123
vitamin K 17

walking 72, 76, 171
water 4
    absorbed in large
        intestine 16
    daily requirements 39
weight gain 154, 169–70
wheat 115, 117, 228
wheat bran 33
withania 27, 171, 193, 205

yeast 47, 64–5
yoga 27, 76
yoghurt 113
    anti-diarrhoeal 94, 95
    choosing 59–60, 61
    dairy sources 60
    homemade 219
    as probiotic 59

zinc 26, 155
    absorption problems
        162, 190
    deficiency 91, 93, 99
    role 161
    sources 162
    supplement 162–3
zinc taste-perception test
    (zinc tally) 123, 161–2